Emergency CT Scans of the Head:
A Practical Atlas

EMERGENCY CT SCANS OF THE HEAD:

A Practical Atlas

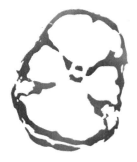

A. ADAM CWINN, MD, FRCPC
Director, Department of Emergency Medicine
Co-Director Trauma Services
Ottawa General Hospital
Associate Professor, Division of Emergency Medicine
University of Ottawa

STEPHEN Z. GRAHOVAC, MD, FRCPC
Neuroradiologist
Ottawa General Hospital
Assistant Professor, Department of Radiology
University of Ottawa

with 338 illustrations

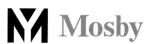

St. Louis   Baltimore   Boston   Carlsbad   Chicago   Minneapolis   New York   Philadelphia   Portland
London   Milan   Sydney   Tokyo   Toronto

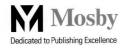

Printed in the United States of America

Mosby–Year Book, Inc.
11830 Westline Industrial Drive
St. Louis, Missouri 63146

Cwinn, A. Adam.
       Emergency CT scans of the head : a practical atlas / A. Adam
Cwinn, Steven Grahovac. — 1st ed.
          p.   cm.
       Includes bibliographical references and index.
       ISBN 0-8151-2621-2
       1. Head—Tomography—Atlases. 2. Medical emergencies—Atlases.
   3. Head—Diseases—Atlases. 4. Head—Wounds and injuries—Atlases.
   I. Grahovac, Steven. II. Title.
       [DNLM: 1. Brain—radiography—atlases. 2. Brain Diseases—
   radiography—atlases. 3. Head Injuries—radiography—atlases.
       4. Tomography, X-Ray Computed—atlases. WL 17 C993e 1998]
   RC936.C86   1998
   617.5 ' 107572—dc21
   DNLM/DLC
                                                                                    97-42384

FORWARD

Confronted with a patient with acute neurologic symptoms in the middle of the night, the frontline troops must be able to interpret a CT scan of the head with the same degree of comfort as a chest radiograph. This atlas is designed to provide assistance in rapid, real time CT scan interpretation. It is intended for use by emergency physicians, general internists, neurologists, general radiologists, radiology technicians, students, and house staff.

Not every conceivable type of CT abnormality could be included—we have tried to balance the number of CT images presented with the practicality of creating a concise book that will be read and used. Only the most relevant frames from each CT study were chosen for reproduction. The important findings are often described in the captions rather than labelled so that the reader can analyse the image as they would in real life. By their nature, CTs have artifacts and those that are commonly encountered are identified. We comment on the clinical abnormalities present for each patient; other areas of the scans that may seem abnormal to the reader represent artifacts or normal anatomic structures.

ACKNOWLEDGEMENTS

Our patients and students have been an inspiration for this work, which will hopefully contribute to the care of patients with neurologic emergencies. Stuart Joyce, your enthusiasm and attention to detail in medical photography made this possible. Our thanks to Garth Dickinson, M.D. for his insightful suggestions. At Mosby, thank you Kathy Falk, Carol Weis, and Florence Achenbach for your guidance and patience.

For our wives and children, this was one more bit of after hours doctoring that took us away from family life and we hope that our love sustained you during the preparation of this work, which we dedicate to you.

A. ADAM CWINN
STEPHEN Z. GRAHOVAC

CONTENTS

Chapter 1 ESSENTIALS OF CT SCANS TO THE HEAD, 1
History of CT, 1
CT versus MRI, 1
Patient postioning, 1
CT physics made easy, 1
Window and level settings, 3
Noncontrast versus contrast cranial CT scans, 4
Analysis of images, 4
Normal CT anatomy, 9
CSF-containing spaces and venous structures, 9

IMAGES, 10
Normal CT anatomy, 16

Chapter 2 TRAUMA, 31

IMAGES
Epidural hematoma, 32
Acute subdural hematoma (SDH), 37
Subacute and chronic SDH, 44
Punctate hemorrhage and contusions, 52
Mixed SDH, contusions, SAH, and miscellaneous injuries, 57

Chapter 3 ISCHEMIC STROKE, 63
Hemorrhagic infarct, 64
Luxury perfusion, 64
Watershed infarctions, 65

IMAGES, 66

Chapter 4 SUBARACHNOID HEMORRHAGE (SAH) AND ANEURYSMS, 85

IMAGES, 88
Subarachnoid hemorrhage, 87
Aneurysms, 98

Chapter 5   NONTRAUMATIC HEMORRHAGE AND VASCULAR MALFORMATIONS, 103

Hypertension, 103
Aneurysms, 103
Vascular malformations (AVMs), 104

IMAGES, 105
Hemorrhage, 105
Ateriovenous malformation (AVM), 110

Chapter 6   INTRACRANIAL NEOPLASMS, 115

Extra-axial tumors, 116
Intra-axial tumors, 116
Tumors of specific areas, 117
Metastases, 119
CT characteristics of tumors, 119

IMAGES, 121

Chapter 7   INTRACRANIAL INFECTIONS, 149

Chronic infections, 149
Parasitic infections, 149
Bacterial infections, 149
Viral infections, 151

IMAGES, 105
Intracranial Infections, 151

Chapter 8   MISCELLANEOUS CONDITIONS, 157

IMAGES, 157
Hydrocephalus/atrophy, 157
Other miscellaneous conditions, 165

Chapter 9   VARIATIONS OF NORMAL STRUCTURES, ARTIFACTS, AND CONGENITAL ABNORMALITIES, 177

Variations of normal structures, 177
Artifacts, 177
Congenital malformations, 178

IMAGES, 181
Vascular structures, 181
Calcifications, 185
Subarachnoid spaces and cisterns, 188
Miscellaneous, 192

EMERGENCY CT SCANS OF THE HEAD:
A Practical Atlas

CHAPTER 1

ESSENTIALS OF CT SCANS OF THE HEAD

History of CT

In 1970, Sir Jeffery Hounsfield combined a mathematical reconstruction formula developed in the 1900s with a rotating combination of x-ray source, detectors, and a computer to produce the first computerized axial tomographic unit, now more commonly known as a CT scanner. For this work he was rewarded a Nobel prize and knighthood. It may be difficult for younger physicians to imagine a world without cross-sectional imaging. The development of this technology truly revolutionized the practice of medicine and accelerated the development of other cross-sectional imaging modalities.

CT Versus MRI

Presently, and for the foreseeable future, CT scanning is the modality of choice for imaging patients with emergency conditions resulting from trauma or other processes that cause acute neurologic compromise. Several factors indicate CT over MRI in the emergency situation, including: (1) availability of CT scanners in nearly all hospitals in the western world, (2) a relatively low cost of CT compared to MRI, and (3) a faster examination time, which allows obtainability of a technically good study in an uncooperative patient.

In distinction to MRI, there are no contraindications for obtaining a CT scan of the head. The patient need only be clinically stable enough to leave the emergency department.

In the emergency evaluation of a patient with suspected stroke, the main diagnostic objective is to rapidly determine disease processes that have caused hemorrhage. CT is superior to MRI in the demonstration of acute hemorrhage. CT also exquisitely demonstrates bony architecture, which is useful in the setting of trauma.

Remember there are some disadvantages of CT versus MRI in the acute setting, the most important of which is poor resolution of pathology in the posterior fossa and brainstem. This is primarily a result of bone artifacts, particularly in the area of the petrous bone.

Patient Positioning

To perform a CT scan of the head, the patient's head is placed in a holder to minimize motion. The patient is moved through the opening in the gantry to obtain the images. The gantry is the circular structure that contains the x-ray source and detectors. The first image to be obtained is a scout view, which resembles a lateral skull x-ray. The scout view is used as a planning aid on which a numbered map is superimposed by the technologist to determine where the image slices will be taken. Then a series of axial images (cross-sectional images in the transverse plane) is obtained from the skull base to the vertex. Most institutions presently angle the gantry and therefore determine the angle of the slices in reference to the orbitomeatal line (a line between the superolateral margin of the orbit and the auditory meatus). Most routine imaging of the adult head is obtained with sequential 10 mm thick axial slices. That is, the entire brain is imaged with no gaps between the slices. Imaging of the posterior fossa usually involves substitution of 5 mm or even 3 mm thick sequential contiguous axial images. These thin slices can also be requested through other regions of the brain to more clearly demonstrate abnormalities.

CT Physics Made Easy

X-rays are absorbed in different degrees by different tissues. This varies from almost no absorption by air to extreme absorption by such tissues such as bone. The density of soft tissues is intermediate between air and bone. On plain x-ray films, soft tissues appear as a relatively homogeneous intermediate density, such as is seen within the cranial vault on a plain lateral skull view. CT is revolutionary because it distinguishes different types of soft tissue on the basis of small differences in the absorption of x-rays. In addition, if visual, qualitative evaluation of the tissue of interest is unclear, a numerical value of the

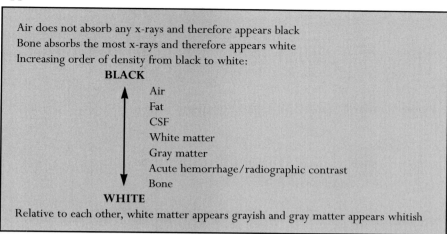

Air does not absorb any x-rays and therefore appears black
Bone absorbs the most x-rays and therefore appears white
Increasing order of density from black to white:

BLACK

Air
Fat
CSF
White matter
Gray matter
Acute hemorrhage/radiographic contrast
Bone

WHITE

Relative to each other, white matter appears grayish and gray matter appears whitish

density can be determined to obtain a quantitative evaluation and hence a precise diagnosis of the type of tissue that is present at a specific location.

Window and Level Settings

The range of tissue densities depicted can be altered by changing the "window settings," and the relative brightness of tissues within a window setting can be changed by altering the "level settings." As an analogy, the volume of a stereo can be adjusted to determine the loudness of a particular segment of music so that various instruments can be heard better (window setting) and at any particular volume the treble can be adjusted to vary the brightness of the sound (level setting). A final clarification: the term *level setting* does not refer to the anatomic position at which the cut is taken; it refers to the relative brightness of the different tissue densities demonstrated by the accompanying window setting.

By changing window and level settings, the appearance of the image can be tailored depending on whether one needs to see very small differences in density of soft tissues or bony anatomy or even the bone soft tissue interface. For instance, a wide window setting of 3000 is used to demonstrate bone pathology. Standard windows for visualizing different densities of brain, blood, and cerebral spinal fluid (CSF) is 80.

Noncontrast Versus Contrast Cranial CT Scans

In the emergency setting, a noncontrast study should be performed first because important information, in particular the presence of acute intracranial hemorrhage, is lost after intravenous contrast enhancement. Contrast can always be administered after the noncontrast study but it is important to remember that the effect of contrast enhancement can not be removed for many hours. Contrast may mask the recognition and delay appropriate treatment of serious conditions such as subarachnoid or intracerebral hemorrhage, subacute infarction, or even encephalitis.

In the trauma patient, the sequence of various imaging studies of other body regions must be carefully planned to not obscure acute intracranial hemorrhage by radiographic contrast administered for the other studies.

Lesions enhance with contrast or appear to abnormally enhance if: (1) the blood-brain barrier is compromised (as occurs with neoplasms and abscesses), allowing the contrast material to leak through the capillaries, and (2) there is increased vascularity and therefore a greater concentration of the dye, for example, (a) AV malformation or aneurysmal sac and (b) a tumor compresses and compacts the normal brain and blood vessels around the perimeter of the lesion.

Analysis of Images

There are many approaches to analysis of a cranial CT scan. We mainly adopt one that works for us individually, but having adopted an approach it is important to stick to it for every scan and analyze the visualized structures on each slice. Failure to look at all the images results in misinterpretations or important findings being missed. As in anything else, there is no substitute for seeing many scans to become proficient.

Every CT scan should be interpreted with the following concepts in mind. They are summarized in the box on page 29 and further illustrated and elaborated upon in subsequent chapters.

1. **Scout View** Perform a brief overview of the scout film to assess the bony architecture at the level of the skull vault, the base of the skull, the upper cervical spine, and the size of the pituitary fossa. In addition, this scout view will often have a legend of the performed axial images posted on it (Figure 1-8, *A*). This legend aids in the precise anatomical localization of normal and abnormal structures.

2. **Mass effect** The presence or absence of mass effect must be determined. Presence or absence could be the result of a space occupying lesion, edema, or a combination of the two. Mass effect is usually diagnosed when there is focal, or often unilateral, effacement (compression) of the ventricles or subarachnoid spaces. *Compression of the subarachnoid spaces results in the effacement of cortical sulci and cisterns.*

3. **Diffuse cerebral edema** If all the cortical sulci, the ventricles, and possibly even the basal cisterns are small, one should consider diffuse cerebral edema as the cause. The inability to clearly identify the basal cisterns also could be the result of a small amount of acute or subacute subarachnoid hemorrhage within these cisterns, or it may indicate the presence of an accompanying tentorial or uncal herniation, usually in the downward but occasionally in the upward direction.

4. **Hydrocephalus** The presence of hydrocephalus is important to recognize and basically is diagnosed when the *ventricles are disproportionately enlarged relative to the cortical sulci.* The temporal horns of the lateral ventricles require careful evaluation because they are the most sensitive indicators of raised intraventricular pressure. The temporal horns are the first structures to enlarge when hydrocephalus is developing.

   If only part of the ventricular system is enlarged, a noncommunicating (also termed *obstructive*) hydrocephalus exists. If the entire ventricular system is dilated, the presence of a communicating (also termed *nonobstructive*) hydrocephalus is suggested. However, an obstructing lesion at the outlet of the fourth ventricle causing a noncommunicating hydrocephalus also can cause dilation of the entire ventricular system.

   Hydrocephalus is caused by an obstruction to the flow of CSF or decreased absorption of CSF. The route of flow of CSF is as follows (and obstruction to flow can occur at any level): the lateral ventricles→ foramina of Monro→third ventricle→aqueduct of Sylvius→fourth ventricle→foramina of Luschka (lateral)/foramen of Magendie (midline)→cisterna magna. The CSF flows from the cisterna magna over the cerebral convexities and is then absorbed through the arachnoid villi into the sagittal sinus, which is a venous structure. Decreased absorption is due to pathology at the level of the arachnoid villi.

- Hydrocephalus is "active" when the intraventricular pressure is raised, causing progressive enlargement of the ventricles.

- Hydrocephalus is "balanced" or "arrested" when compensatory mechanisms allow the intraventricular pressure to return to normal so that the ventricles no longer tend to enlarge.

In severe or active hydrocephalus the cortical sulci are effaced (compressed). Another feature suggesting that the intraventricular pressure is raised is blunting of the margins of the ventricular system. This is most pronounced in the area of the temporal horns and these structures appear "ballooned." When the hydrocephalus is active in nature there is also evidence of finger-like hypodensities adjacent to the frontal and occipital horns that result from *transependymal flow* of CSF.

5. **Atrophy**   Atrophy is a common finding on many CT scans performed in a busy emergency department because the incidence of neurologic symptoms increases with increasing age. Confusion sometimes exists in differentiating the ventricular enlargement associated with cerebral atrophy from hydrocephalus. In general, *cerebral atrophy produces enlargement of the cortical sulci and subarachnoid cisterns. This may result in passive, compensatory enlargement of the ventricular system.*
    Cerebral atrophy is composed of varying proportions of cortical and subcortical atrophy. *Cortical atrophy* is predominantly atrophy of the gray matter at the surface of the brain. *Subcortical atrophy* is predominantly atrophy of the white matter located beneath the cortex. Generally, cortical atrophy is associated with sulcal enlargement and subcortical atrophy is associated with ventricular enlargement; however, both areas are invariably enlarged to a greater or lesser degree.
    Remember that in hydrocephalus *there is disproportionate enlargement of the ventricular system relative to the cortical sulci and subarachnoid cisterns.*

6. **Cerebral infarction**   The presence of a cerebral infarction is often not evident on CT in the first 12 to 24 hours. However, early in the course of infarction, subtle mass effect may be appreciated in the area of involvement and this usually manifests as sulcal effacement (compres-

sion). Loss of the normal gray-white differentiation frequently can be seen in the area of involvement. This is seen earliest in the area of the insular cortex in cases of middle cerebral artery infarction and is colloquially termed "loss of the insular stripe." In addition, one may detect hyperdense acute thrombus in the affected artery well before the secondary signs of cerebral infarction are evident.

7. **Midline and subtle abnormalities** It is relatively easy to spot a localized or a unilateral abnormality. However, diffuse abnormalities and abnormalities involving the midline structures, which are unpaired and therefore have no counterpart for visual comparison, are most easily missed or misinterpreted. For this reason an atlas or a normal CT scan should be available in the emergency department for comparison purposes.

8. **Abnormal hyperdensities** Remember that hyperdensities appear white and the degree of whiteness depends on the density of the tissues and determines the type of tissue one is seeing, such as acute hemorrhage, calcification, or ossification.

    Calcification or ossification should have the same density appearance as the skull vault when window and level adjustments are optimized for bony detail.

    Acute hemorrhage is not visible on bony windows; it is seen only on soft tissue windows after clot retraction and it appears increasingly hyperdense in proportion to the amount of hemorrhage. The precise *localization* of the hemorrhage must then be determined, i.e., is it intra-axial within the brain parenchyma or extra-axial within the ventricles, subarachnoid, subdural, or epidural spaces? Subdural hemorrhage is hyperdense acutely, appears isodense between five to ten days after the ictus, and hypodense after approximately ten days.

    Intravenously administered contrast *medium* is also hyperdense. It appears approximately as dense (white) as blood clot appears on soft tissue windows.

9. **Abnormal hypodensities (low density changes)** Remember that hypodensities appear dark and the degree of darkness depends on the density of the tissues and determines the type of abnormality one is seeing. The following hypodensities may be encountered.

   - Air and Gas
     The most extreme hypodensities are caused by air or gas products. The presence of air intracranially is abnormal and a search for its

cause is warranted if there is no history of recent lumbar puncture or craniotomy. Air collections usually appear as small droplets located in the subarachnoid or subdural space. They are often adjacent to a fracture of the skull vault or skull base. Intracranial air associated with basilar skull fractures is due to communication with the mastoid air cells or paranasal sinuses.

Intracranial gas collections result from gas producing microorganisms associated with cerebral abscesses and are quite rare. This gas cannot be distinguished from air collections on CT.

- Fat
  Fat appears similar to air on the CT scan but if one were to actually measure its attenuation coefficient it would be higher than air. This can be done practically to assist with the diagnosis. Intracranial fat collections are abnormal and usually associated with benign tumors such as lipomas or dermoids. Dermoids have a tendency to rupture and spread their contents, in the form of fat droplets, throughout the subarachnoid space, frequently inciting a chemical meningitis.

- Gray Matter Hypodensities
  Cerebral infarctions, after approximately 12 to 24 hours, produce hypodense change in the involved gray matter. Recall that there is gray matter in the cortex and the basal ganglia and either region may exhibit hypodense changes with infarction. Because healthy white matter is normally hypodense (darker) compared to healthy gray matter, when infarction causes the gray matter to become hypodense, it produces a so-called *"loss of differentiation of the gray-white interface."* When cerebral infarctions become chronic there is further decrease in density as encephalomalacia develops.

- White Matter Hypodensities
  Low density change confined to the white matter often has a "finger-like" configuration. This is usually the result of disease processes that cause white matter edema or, less commonly, white matter ischemia such as is seen with leukomalacia secondary to small vessel angiopathy or radiation treatment. There may be local mass effect associated with white matter edema. Further investigation of an underlying cause for this is most conveniently performed with a contrast enhanced CT scan.

- Tumors

  Before contrast enhancement most tumors are predominantly iso-dense to white matter and are slightly hypodense to normal gray matter. Therefore tumors within white matter may be difficult to appreciate on a nonenhanced CT. Although most tumors are associated with blood-brain barrier disruption and consequent contrast enhancement, low grade tumors, particularly low grade gliomas show no change in appearance after the administration of contrast media.

Normal CT Anatomy

Familiarity with some normal neuroanatomy is necessary for interpretation of CT scans. The images at the end of this chapter cover the essential knowledge base of normal structures as they appear on a noncontrast and on a contrast enhanced CT scan. The reader is strongly encouraged to study these images before proceeding to the images in subsequent chapters. It is always useful to come back to these images of normal CT anatomy if one is puzzled by a finding on a patient's scan or on one of the images in the subsequent chapters.

Some understanding of the CSF-containing spaces, venous drainage, and arterial circulation is needed before proceeding to the normal scans.

CSF-Containing Spaces and Venous Structures

On a noncontrast CT scan, the CSF-containing structures (cisterns and ventricles) have a hypodense appearance. Many important and larger cerebral arteries and veins course through the subarachnoid space and can be identified because of the hypodensity that surrounds these vascular structures.

It is necessary to be familiar with the anatomy of the CSF-containing spaces and the venous structures to interpret CT scans correctly. Figures 1-1 to 1-5 should be reviewed carefully.

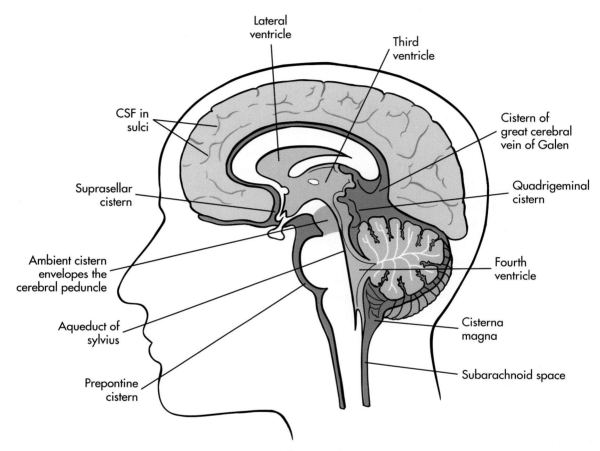

FIGURE 1-1 Basal cisterns, lateral view.

A

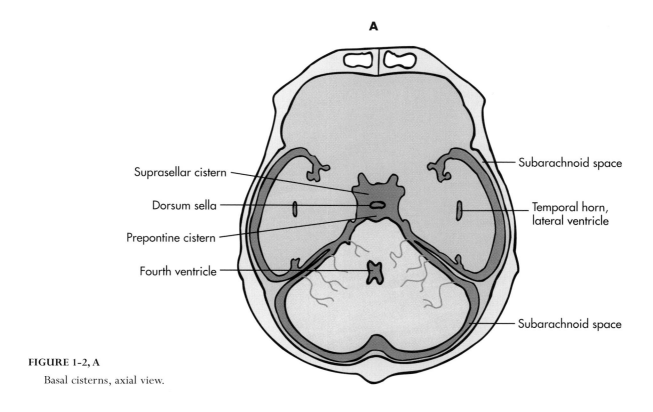

Suprasellar cistern

Dorsum sella

Prepontine cistern

Fourth ventricle

Subarachnoid space

Temporal horn, lateral ventricle

Subarachnoid space

FIGURE 1-2, A

Basal cisterns, axial view.

B

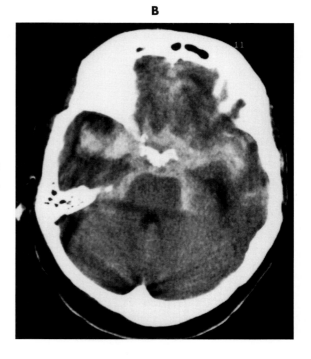

FIGURE 1-2, B

Basal cisterns, axial view. This noncontrast CT of a patient with a large subarachnoid hemorrhage compliments Figure 1-3, A, by demonstrating blood in the basilar cisterns.

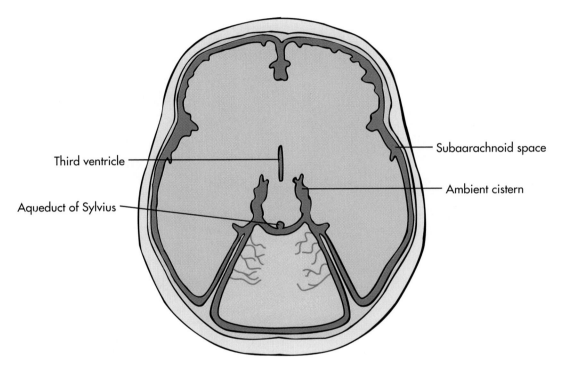

Third ventricle

Aqueduct of Sylvius

Subaarachnoid space

Ambient cistern

FIGURE 1-3 Basal cisterns, axial view.

Major Cerebral Veins and Venous Sinuses

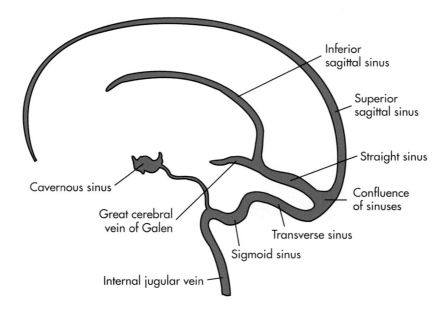

FIGURE 1-4 Lateral view.

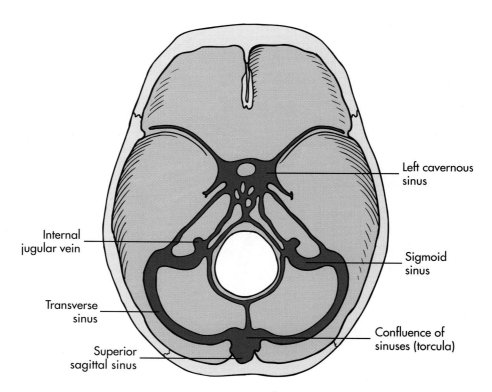

Left cavernous
sinus

Internal
jugular vein

Sigmoid
sinus

Transverse
sinus

Confluence of
sinuses (torcula)

Superior
sagittal sinus

FIGURE 1-5 Axial view.

Arterial Supply and Vascular Territories

With the rapid developments in the treatment of stroke an understanding of the arterial supply and vascular territories of the brain is useful and essential for the interpretation of CT findings in cases of infarction. To this end, Figures 1-6 and 1-7 will hopefully be of value.

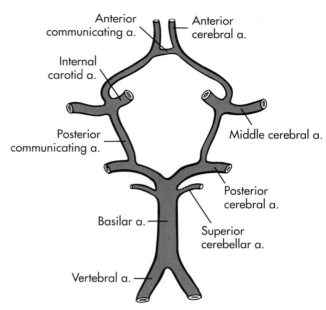

FIGURE 1-6 Circle of Willis.

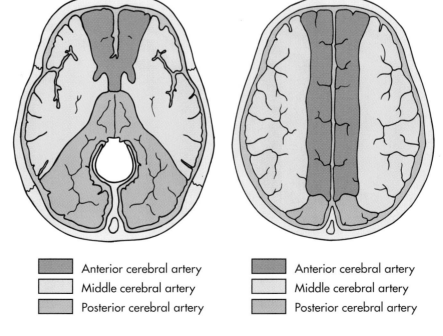

FIGURE 1-7 Arterial vascular territories.

Anterior cerebral artery
Middle cerebral artery
Posterior cerebral artery

Anterior cerebral artery
Middle cerebral artery
Posterior cerebral artery

Normal CT Anatomy

The following images provide the essential normal anatomy of the brain on axial CT imaging (Figures 1-8 to 1-10).

Normal Young Adult • (Noncontrast)

FIGURE 1-8, A-O

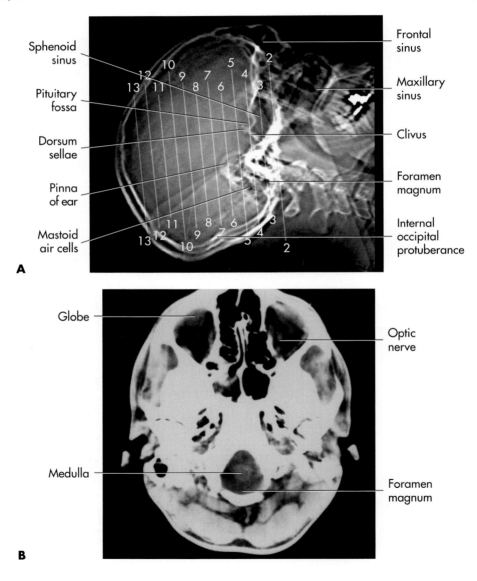

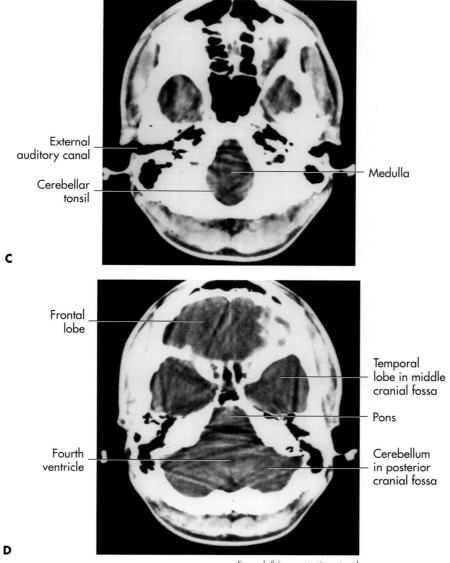

C

External auditory canal

Cerebellar tonsil

Medulla

Frontal lobe

Temporal lobe in middle cranial fossa

Pons

Fourth ventricle

Cerebellum in posterior cranial fossa

D

Figure 1-8 (noncontrast) continued

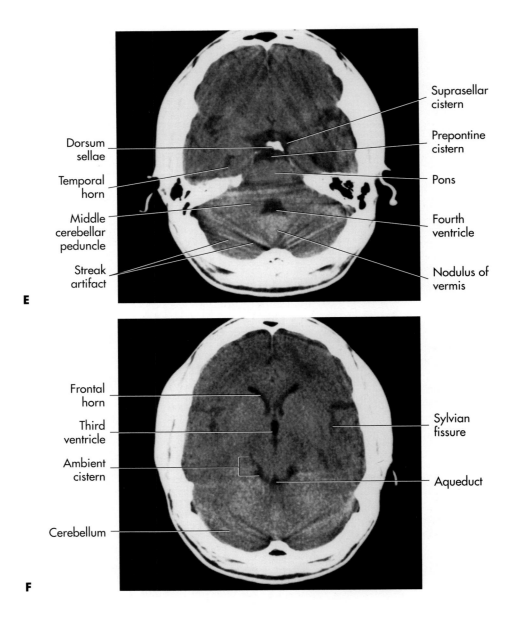

Suprasellar cistern

Prepontine cistern

Pons

Fourth ventricle

Nodulus of vermis

Dorsum sellae

Temporal horn

Middle cerebellar peduncle

Streak artifact

E

Frontal horn

Third ventricle

Ambient cistern

Cerebellum

Sylvian fissure

Aqueduct

F

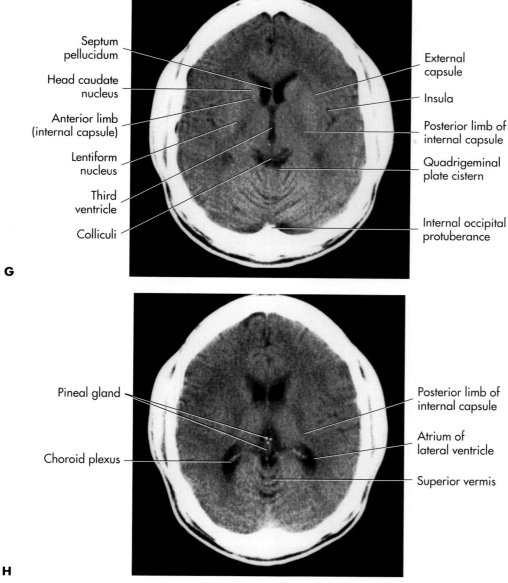

Septum
pellucidum

Head caudate
nucleus

Anterior limb
(internal capsule)

Lentiform
nucleus

Third
ventricle

Colliculi

External
capsule

Insula

Posterior limb of
internal capsule

Quadrigeminal
plate cistern

Internal occipital
protuberance

G

Pineal gland

Choroid plexus

Posterior limb of
internal capsule

Atrium of
lateral ventricle

Superior vermis

H

Figure 1-8 (noncontrast) continued

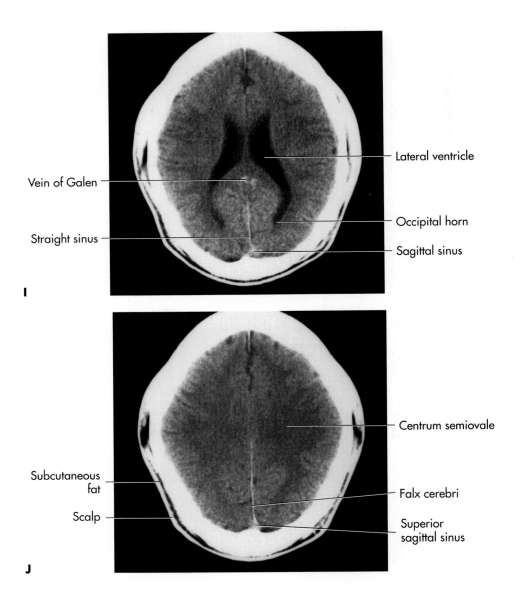

Vein of Galen

Straight sinus

Lateral ventricle

Occipital horn

Sagittal sinus

I

Subcutaneous fat

Scalp

Centrum semiovale

Falx cerebri

Superior sagittal sinus

J

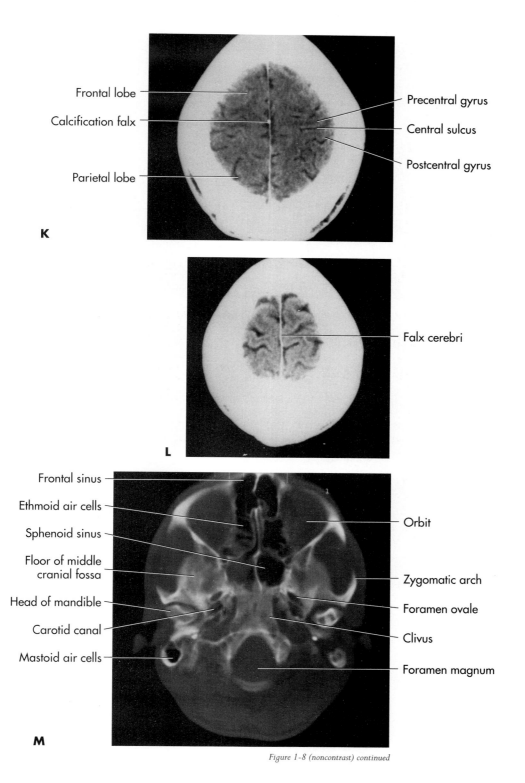

Frontal lobe — Precentral gyrus

Calcification falx — Central sulcus

— Postcentral gyrus

Parietal lobe —

K

L — Falx cerebri

Frontal sinus —
Ethmoid air cells —
Sphenoid sinus — — Orbit
Floor of middle cranial fossa —
Head of mandible — — Zygomatic arch
Carotid canal — — Foramen ovale
— Clivus
Mastoid air cells — — Foramen magnum

M

Figure 1-8 (noncontrast) continued

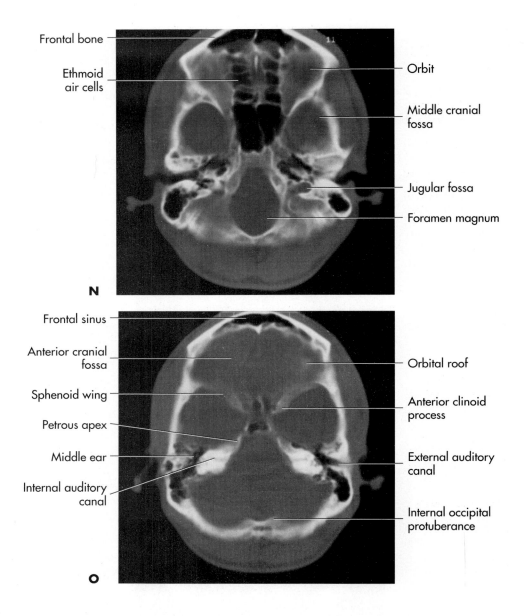

Frontal bone

Ethmoid air cells

Orbit

Middle cranial fossa

Jugular fossa

Foramen magnum

N

Frontal sinus

Anterior cranial fossa

Sphenoid wing

Petrous apex

Middle ear

Internal auditory canal

Orbital roof

Anterior clinoid process

External auditory canal

Internal occipital protuberance

O

Normal Middle-aged Adult • (Noncontrast)

FIGURE 1-9, A–E

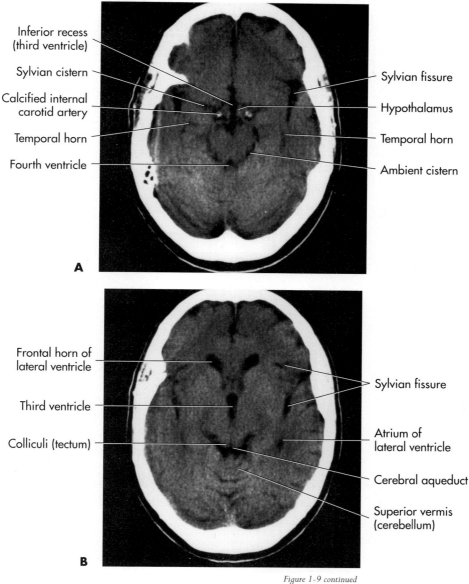

Inferior recess (third ventricle)
Sylvian cistern
Calcified internal carotid artery
Temporal horn
Fourth ventricle

Sylvian fissure
Hypothalamus
Temporal horn
Ambient cistern

A

Frontal horn of lateral ventricle
Third ventricle
Colliculi (tectum)

Sylvian fissure
Atrium of lateral ventricle
Cerebral aqueduct
Superior vermis (cerebellum)

B

Figure 1-9 continued

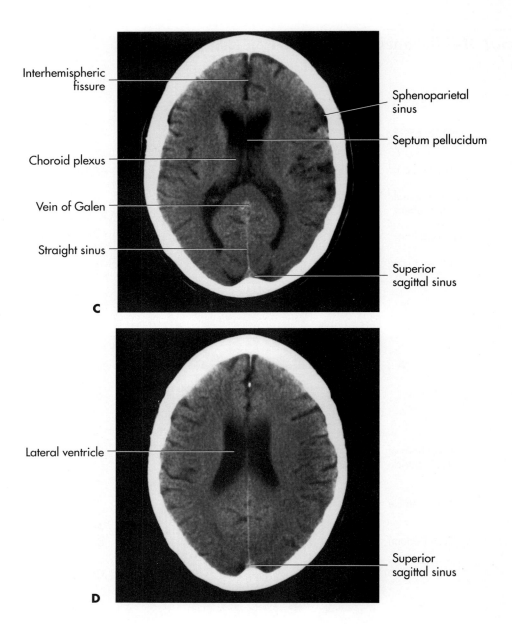

Interhemispheric fissure

Sphenoparietal sinus

Septum pellucidum

Choroid plexus

Vein of Galen

Straight sinus

Superior sagittal sinus

C

Lateral ventricle

Superior sagittal sinus

D

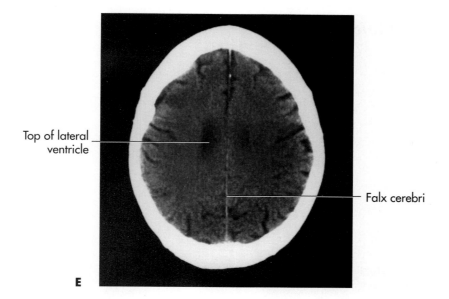

Top of lateral ventricle

Falx cerebri

E

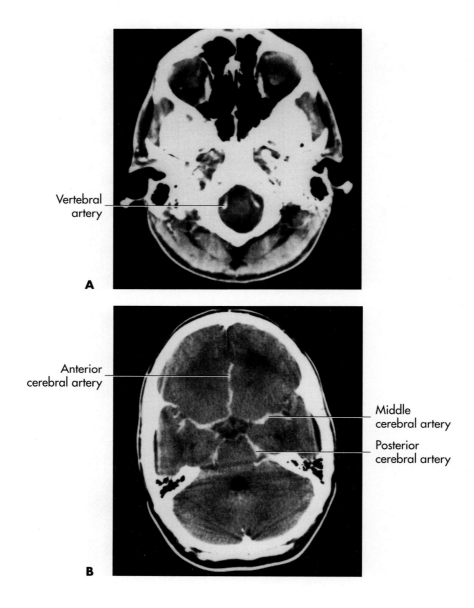

Vertebral
artery

A

Anterior
cerebral artery

Middle
cerebral artery

Posterior
cerebral artery

B

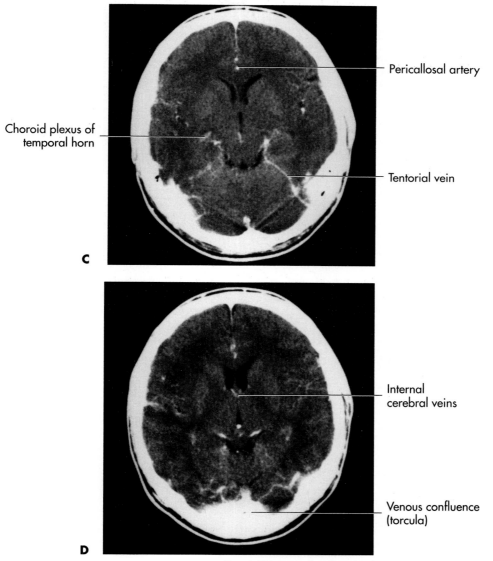

Pericallosal artery

Choroid plexus of
temporal horn

Tentorial vein

C

Internal
cerebral veins

Venous confluence
(torcula)

D

Figure 1-10 (contrast-enhanced) continued

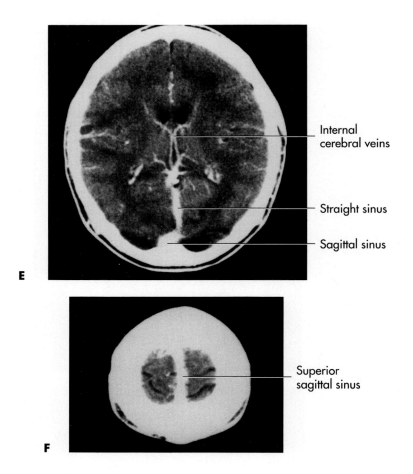

Internal
cerebral veins

Straight sinus

Sagittal sinus

E

Superior
sagittal sinus

F

The points in the box below will be discussed further in subsequent chapters. They should be answered mentally in every CT interpretation.

Checklist for Interpreting CT of the Head

1. Is there evidence of hemorrhage?
   Is it extra-axial:
      within ventricles?
      within subdural space?
      within subarachnoid space?
      within epidural space?
   Is it intra-axial and, if so, in what area of the brain parenchyma?
2. Is there mass effect?
   (local mass effect results in effacement of sulci)
3. Is there diffuse cerebral edema?
   This is suggested by:
      small ventricles
      small basilar cisterns
      general effacement of the cortical sulci
      diffuse loss of the gray-white differentiation
4. Is there local loss of gray-white differentiation?
   Caused by: infarction, tumor, inflammation
5. Is there hydrocephalus?
   Is it communicating or noncommunicating?
6. Have the cisterns been scrutinized for hemorrhage and size?
7. Is there evidence of infarction?
8. Is there calcification?
   Is this in areas of the brain that become calcified? physiologically?
   Is this abnormal calcification?
9. Have the midline structures been examined carefully?
10. Have all the images been analyzed?
      including the scout view and bone windows?
12. Will contrast infusion help elucidate the diagnosis?
13. Is my interpretation of the CT consistent with the clinical findings?

CHAPTER 2

TRAUMA

As opposed to other chapters, very little introduction is required for this topic. Remember that acute hemorrhage is hyperdense (white) on a non-contrast CT.

Epidural hematomas are caused by extra-axial arterial bleeding. Subdural hematomas are caused by venous bleeding of the veins bridging the sub-dural space.

Cerebral contusions will vary in appearance depending on the magnitude of trauma and the interval between injury and scanning. Some small contusions will be visible only as edema and not hemorrhage.

Traumatic subarachnoid hemorrhage (SAH) has the CT features of SAH in general (discussed in Chapter 4).

Skull fractures, facial fractures, and cervical fractures may be seen on the scout view, and this image should always be examined for useful information. Skull fractures are best visualized on the bone windows. Facial and cervical fractures require special CT imaging protocols.

The key features of the CT in a trauma patient are explained in the captions and labelled images that follow.

Epidural Hematoma

Patient 2-1 • **Classic acute epidural hematoma (R temporal)**

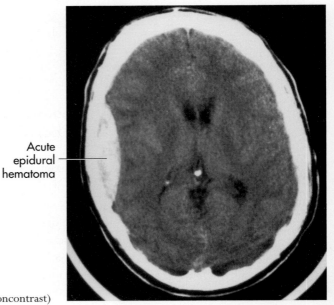

Acute
epidural —
hematoma

FIGURE 2-1 (Noncontrast)

Patient 2-2 • **Large epidural hematoma (L)**

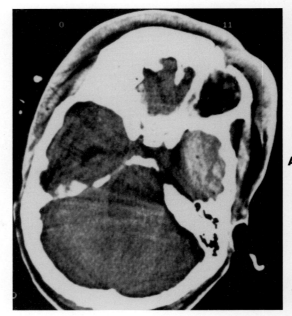

A

FIGURE 2-2, A (Noncontrast)

Epidural hematoma in the left middle cranial fossa with a tiny air bubble in the center suggesting a basal skull fracture.

Rostrocaudal Herniation: Obliteration of the ambient cisterns and the fourth ventricle indicates herniation. There is dilatation of the right temporal horn due to the obstructive hydrocephalus.

FIGURE 2-2, B (Noncontrast)

Swirl Sign: The hematoma has swirls of hypodensity within the hyperdense clot. Blood is hyperdense only when the clot retracts. The hypodense area is caused by brisk bleeding of blood that has not had time to clot. The swirl sign indicates brisk bleeding and that surgery is even more urgent.

The hematoma extends between the coronal and the lambdoidal suture and down to the middle cranial fossa.

RULE: Epidurals never cross suture lines but do cross the midline. On the other hand, subdurals cross suture lines but never cross the midline.

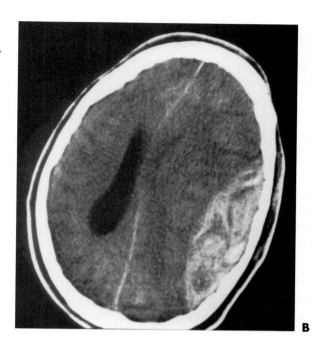

B

FIGURE 2-2, C (Noncontrast)

There is an oblique skull fracture at the base involving the left sphenoid and temporal bones and extending into the base of the pituitary fossa. It likely traverses the foramen spinosum through which courses the middle meningeal artery, which can tear at this level to create the epidural hematoma.

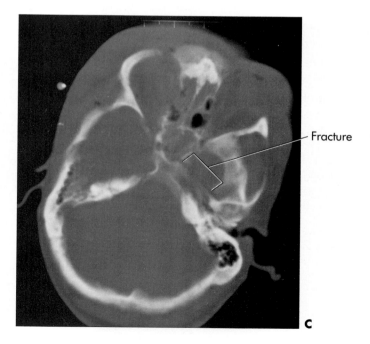

Fracture

C

Patient 2-3 • Subtle epidural hematoma (R temporal)

FIGURE 2-3, A (Noncontrast)

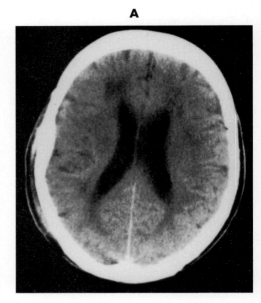

Follow the contour of the inner table of the skull bone. You will notice a slight inward bulge in the right temporal region that is the epidural hematoma. It appears as the same density as bone due to a narrow window level (W80) and might lead one to believe that it is simply an irregularity in the shape of the skull.

Clues to Diagnosis:

1. Pattern recognition after having seen this example of subtle convexity at the inner table.

2. Confirm the abnormality on the cut just above or just below the one in question. The bulge on the cut below in this patient looked exactly the same but is not reproduced to save space.

3. If still in doubt, ask the CT technician to bring the images up on the screen. Adjust the windows until there is a better definition of the abnormality. This was done for this patient (in this case W200) and Figure 2-3, *B*, clearly shows a tiny lens-shaped epidural and a scalp hematoma.

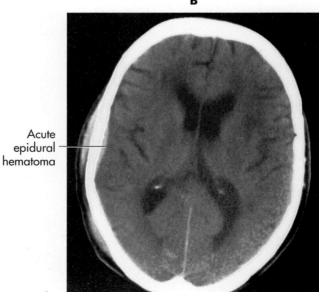

Acute epidural hematoma

FIGURE 2-3, B (Noncontrast)

Patient 2-4 • Epidural hematoma (L frontal)

FIGURE 2-4 (Noncontrast)

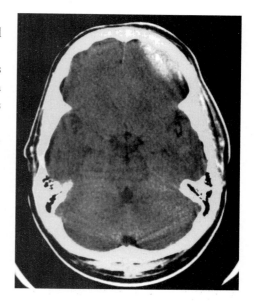

Differential diagnosis: With a history of trauma—epidural hematoma, large contusion, or intraparenchymal bleed.

Why is this an epidural hematoma? (1) The hyperdensity is confluent with the inner table of the skull, and (2) there is a sharp angle at the outer perimeter of the clot where it adjoins the skull.

Note that there is streak artifact from the lesser wing of the sphenoid that tends to take away from the classic appearance of epidural hematoma. Although this is an unusual location for an epidural hematoma, it is important to make the correct diagnosis because this lesion is amenable to surgery whereas contusions are not. If one were not sure, examination of the images with different windows or rescanning with thin cuts through this area might clarify the diagnosis.

Patient 2-5 • Occipital epidural hematoma (R)
• Focal contusion with surrounding edema (R frontal)

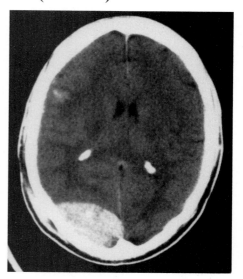

FIGURE 2-5 (Noncontrast)

Patient 2-6 • Acute epidural hematoma in the middle cranial fossa (an unusual location)

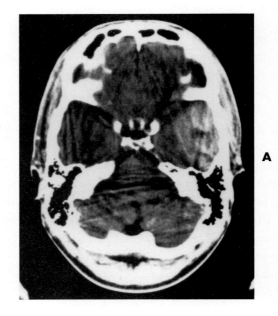

A

FIGURE 2-6, A (Noncontrast)

The following features point to the diagnosis of acute epidural hematoma:

1. Relatively homogeneous hyperdensity
2. No surrounding edema of the brain
3. Lens shaped

B

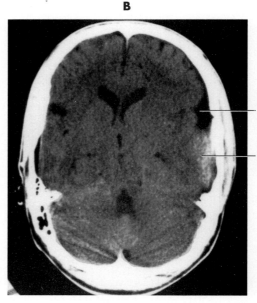

Widened subarachnoid space

Epidural hematoma

FIGURE 2-6, B (Noncontrast)

Noteworthy Point: The extra-axial widening of the subarachnoid space (in this case, in the area of the Sylvian fissure adjacent to the epidural hematoma) is a typical finding with extra-axial masses.

Acute Subdural Hematoma (SDH)

Patient 2-7 • **Acute SDH extending from the frontal region to the temporal parietal region and layering above the tentorium (L)**

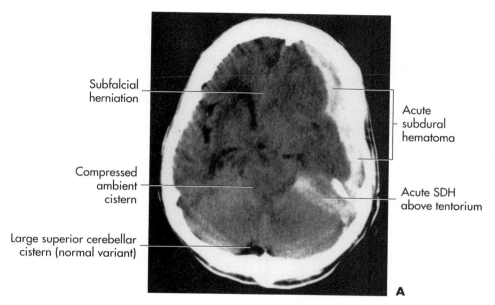

FIGURE 2-7, A (Noncontrast)

Subdural hematomas cross the suture lines (in this case, the coronal and lambdoidal sutures).

Appreciate the loss of sulci adjacent to the subdural due to *local* mass effect as compared to the other side. Contrast this finding with Figure 2-1.

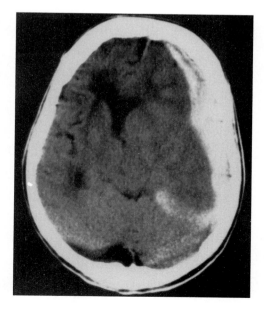

FIGURE 2-7, B

Patient 2-8 • Subtle acute SDH (R temporal parietal)

This may be, in fact, the most subtle subdural hematoma in history. There is a very faint and tiny inhomogeneous hyperdense rim at the right temporal region compared to the left. Even if this was not perceived, there are other findings that should lead you to suspect the diagnosis.

1. The main clue is that on the left-hand side, the sulci are very clearly seen adjacent to the inner table of the skull in the temporal region. On the right side they are indistinct. This is due to the local mass effect of the SDH.
2. On the left-hand side, the Sylvian fissure is clearly seen. On the right-hand side, the Sylvian fissure is smaller (compressed) due to local mass effect.
3. The eye is immediately drawn to the asymmetry of the lateral ventricles. This finding could be a variation of normal or could be due to compression of the lateral ventricle. In context of the other findings, this asymmetry is due to the SDH.
4. Persistence of these findings on other cuts adjacent to the one reproduced here was consistent with the diagnosis.

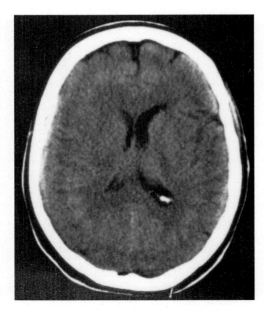

FIGURE 2-8 (Noncontrast)

Patient 2-9 • Acute subdural hematoma below the tentorium in the posterior fossa on the left side

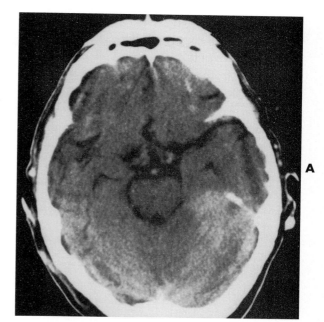

A

FIGURE 2-9, A (Noncontrast)

The tentorium cerebelli normally appears slightly hyperdense (see Figure 2-11). In this case, however, there is significantly increased density on the left in the posterior fossa overlying the left cerebellar hemisphere. This finding should not be ascribed to the normal appearance of the tentorium because it is an acute subdural hematoma below the tentorium. The adjacent cut confirms the pathology.

FIGURE 2-9, B (Noncontrast)

A more highly localized hyperdense area just posterior to the left quadrigeminal plate cistern, which at first glance might be interpreted as a contusion, is clearly confluent with the subdural blood seen on the lower cut in Figure 2-9, *A*.

Noteworthy Point: In general, it may be difficult to decide if the hematoma is above or below the tentorium but it is at least essential to recognize that there is a subdural hematoma in the vicinity of the tentorium. The main clue that this particular SDH is in the posterior fossa is to recognize that the majority of the blood is at the level of the cerebellum, not the occipital lobe, but this can be confirmed with coronal sections if necessary. Be sure to contrast this case with Figures 2-10, *A* and *B*, which is an acute subdural hematoma above the tentorium.

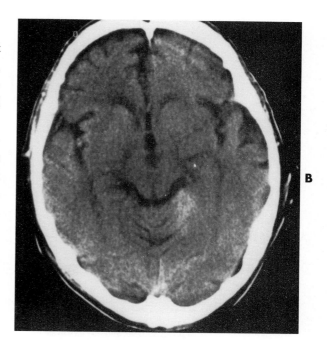

B

Patient 2-10 • Acute SDH layering just above the tentorium (R)

The normal tentorium is often seen at the level of this cut and in fact is visible on the left-hand side as a faint hyperdensity. However, on the right there is a crescent shaped hyperdensity that is too wide and too hyperdense to simply be the tentorium—it is an acute subdural hematoma. It is continuous with the wedge shaped hyperdensity in Figure 2-10, *B*, which extends almost to the midline, providing some evidence that this is above the tentorium. This was confirmed on MRI, Figure 2-10, *C*.

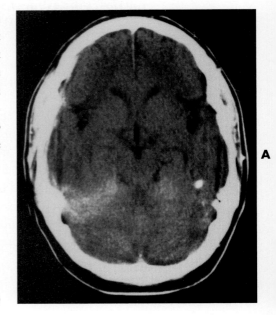

A

FIGURE 2-10, A (Noncontrast)

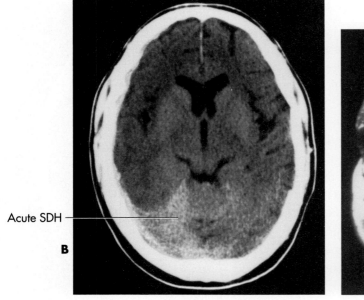

Acute SDH

B

FIGURE 2-10, B (Noncontrast)

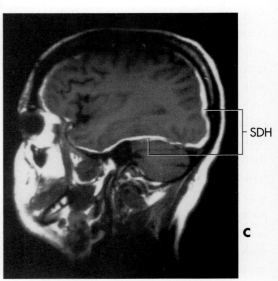

SDH

C

FIGURE 2-10, C (MRI)

Patient 2-11 • Normal CT with normal tentorium and streak artifact from internal occipital protuberance

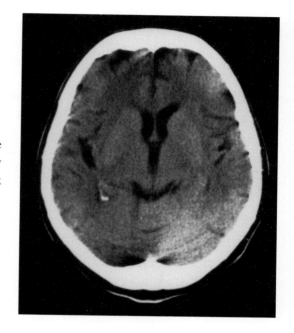

FIGURE 2-11 (Noncontrast)

Compare this normal image with the SDH at the tentorium, Patients 9 and 10. This cut is directly through the normal tentorium on the left. Also, streak artifact is very common in this region.

Patient 2-12 • Occipital acute SDH with intracranial air (L)

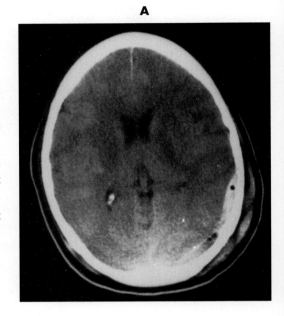

A

FIGURE 2-12, A (Noncontrast)

The subdural hematoma almost appears crescent shaped to suggest an epidural hematoma but this hypothesis is rejected when one examines the cuts at the next higher level (Figure 2-12, *B*).

There are three hypodense air bubbles resulting from a basal skull fracture through the mastoid air cells that was visible on the bone windows but could not be reproduced. On this cut there is also some streak artifact from the internal occipital protuberance.

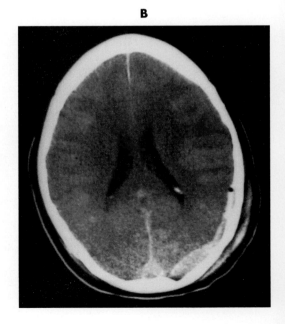

B

FIGURE 2-12, B (Noncontrast)

The SDH crosses the lambdoidal suture. One intracranial air bubble is seen.

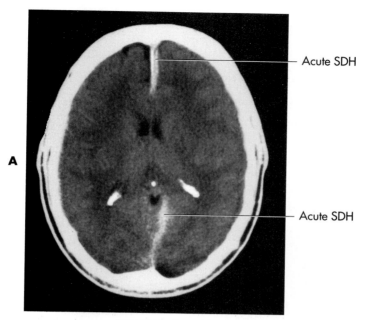

A   Acute SDH

Acute SDH

FIGURE 2-13, A (Noncontrast)

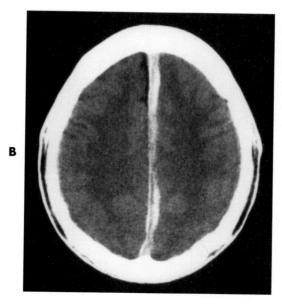

B

FIGURE 2-13, B (Noncontrast)

Subacute and Chronic SDH

Noteworthy Points:

- Acute SDH appears hyperdense
- Subacute SDH appears isodense (approximately 5-10 days after bleed)
- Chronic SDH appears hypodense (approximately 10 days or more after bleed)

Patient 2-14 • **Subacute SDH (L)**

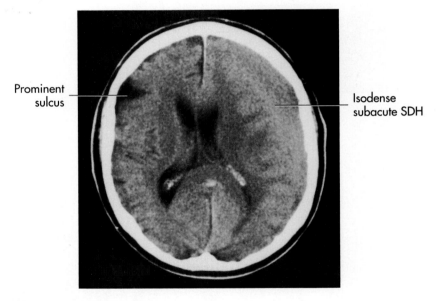

Prominent sulcus

Isodense subacute SDH

FIGURE 2-14 (Noncontrast)
Isodense SDH with midline shift to right and subfalcial herniation.

Patient 2-15 • Acute on chronic SDH (R)

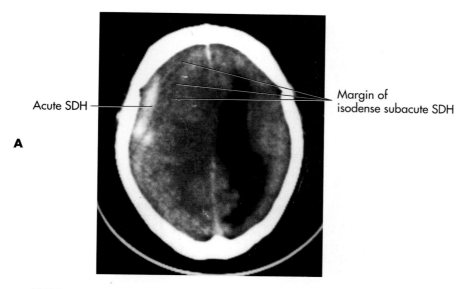

Acute SDH —

Margin of
isodense subacute SDH

A

FIGURE 2-15, A (Noncontrast)

Right lateral ventricle is obliterated from compression. Subfalcial herniation to the left. Left ventricle prominent due to obstructive hydrocephalus.

FIGURE 2-15, B (Contrast enhanced)

The chronic SDH has compressed the meningeal vasculature along the right cerebral cortex, which enhances with contrast and outlines the extent of the chronic SDH.

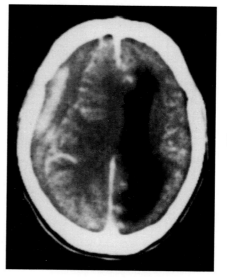

B

Patient 2-16 • Chronic SDH (R frontal) and acute SDH (R tentorium) and posterior falx

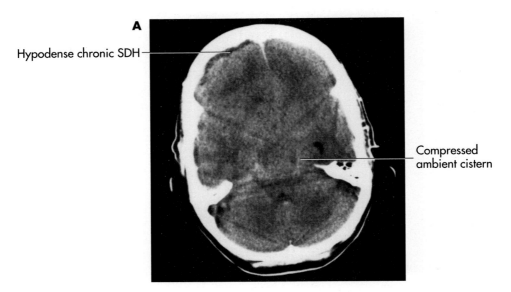

Hypodense chronic SDH

Compressed ambient cistern

FIGURE 2-16, A (Noncontrast)
Ambient cistern compressed.

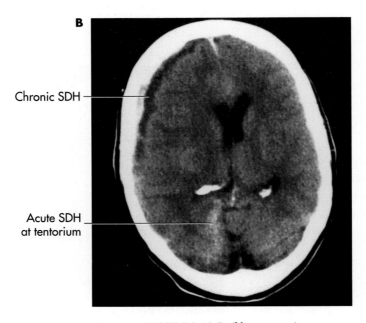

Chronic SDH

Acute SDH at tentorium

FIGURE 2-16, B (Noncontrast)

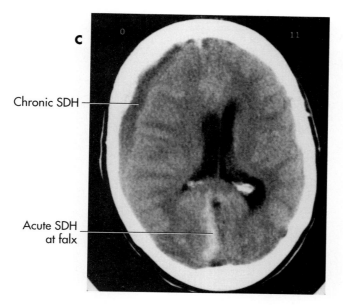

Chronic SDH —

Acute SDH —
at falx

FIGURE 2-16, C (Noncontrast)

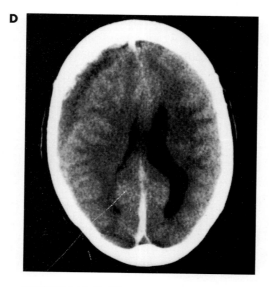

FIGURE 2-16, D (Noncontrast)
Acute SDH posterior falx and chronic SDH (R frontal)

Patient 2-17 • **Chronic SDH (bilateral)**

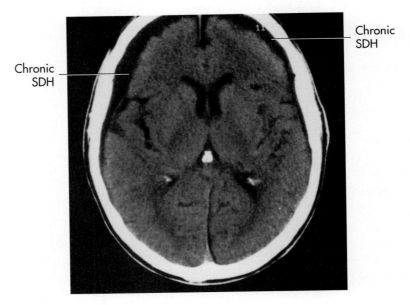

Chronic
SDH

Chronic
SDH

FIGURE 2-17 (Noncontrast)

Why isn't this atrophy? Generally, a prominent subarachnoid space associated with atrophy also has associated adjacent large cortical sulci. In distinction, this case demonstrates a large subdural space with small adjacent cortical sulci, as would be expected with a SDH.

Patient 2-18 • Chronic SDH (L frontoparietal) with subfalcial herniation

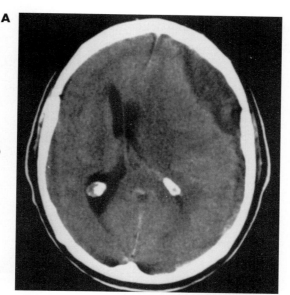

FIGURE 2-18, A   (Noncontrast)

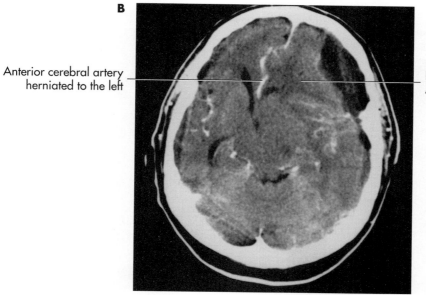

Anterior cerebral artery
herniated to the left

Ischemia in
ACA territory

FIGURE 2-18, B (Contrast enhanced)
    Note that the SDH has caused herniation of
the anterior cerebral artery (ACA), causing subcortical ischemia in that territory.

Patient 2-19 • Acute on chronic SDH with fluid/fluid level (R frontoparietal)

FIGURE 2-19 (Noncontrast)

The red blood cells form the acute component of the hemorrhage layer in the dependant position (hematocrit effect).

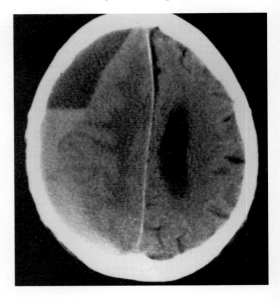

Patient 2-20 • Chronic SDH (R)

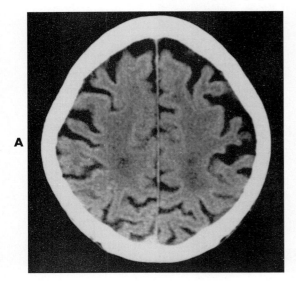

A

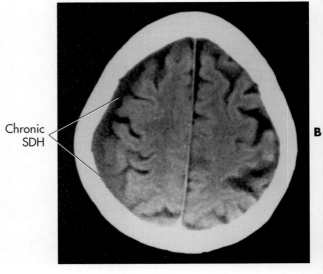

Chronic
SDH

B

FIGURE 2-20, A (Noncontrast)

After a head injury, this patient had a normal CT scan except for atrophy.

FIGURE 2-20, B (Noncontrast)

The same patient had this CT scan two months later showing a chronic SDH of the frontoparietal area (R). Note the smaller size of the gyri ipsilaterally due to local mass effect from the SDH.

Patient 2-21 • Chronic SDH (Bilateral)

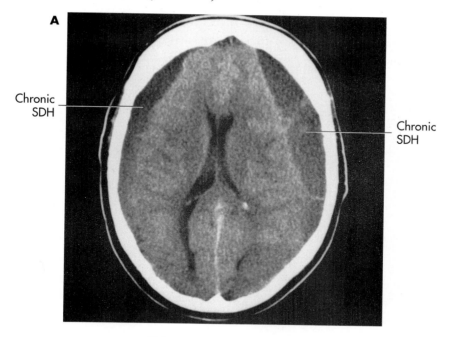

Chronic SDH

Chronic SDH

FIGURE 2-21, A (Noncontrast)

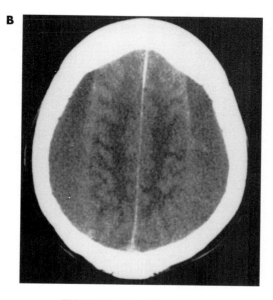

FIGURE 2-21, B (Noncontrast)

Punctate Hemorrhage and Contusions

Patient 2-22 • Occipital fracture and contrecoup punctate hemorrhage and diffuse axonal injury

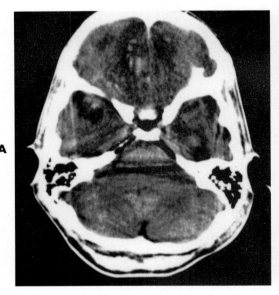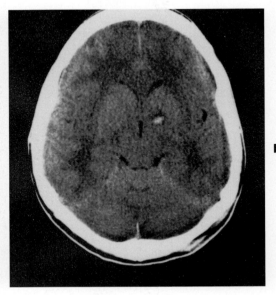

FIGURE 2-22, A (Noncontrast)

Punctate hemorrhagic contusions in the frontal lobes and middle cranial fossae on both sides. The marked hypodensity surrounding the contusions is edema.

FIGURE 2-22, B (Noncontrast)

There is a focal punctate hyperdensity in the left basal ganglia consistent with focal contusion. This can be distinguished from a commonly seen variation of normal, calcification in the basal ganglia, based on the fact that the hyperdensity is not quite as dense as bone and there is clearly some surrounding hypodensity, which signifies edema (see Figure 3-3 for comparison of normal calcification within the basal ganglia). Also note the normal tentorium cerebelli on the left and right sides.

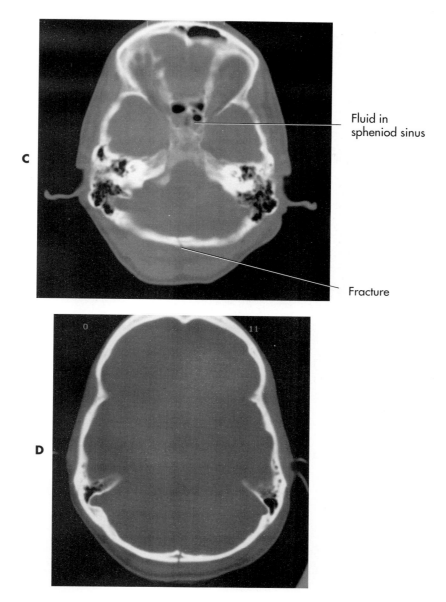

C

Fluid in
spheniod sinus

Fracture

D

FIGURE 2-22, C and D (Bone windows)

A linear fracture is seen in the midline. Remember that the sagittal suture stops at the level of a higher cut. There is also fluid in the sphenoid sinus.

Patient 2-23 • Bifrontal contusions and acute hemorrhage in the intrahemispheric fissure

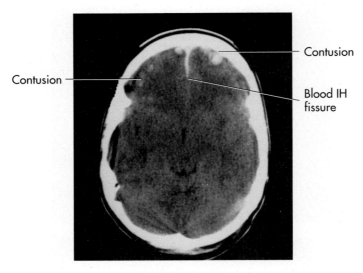

FIGURE 2-23 (Noncontrast)

Patient 2-24 • Frontal contusion (R)

FIGURE 2-24 (Noncontrast)

Noteworthy Point: Effacement of sulci on the right is due to local mass effect from edema. Differential diagnosis in the absence of a history of trauma is infection, tumor, intracerebral hemorrhage, and hemorrhagic infarction.

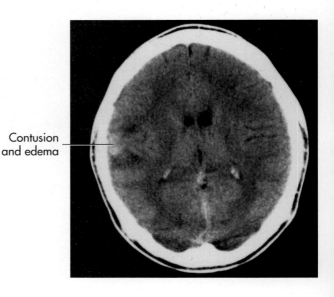

Patient 2-25 • Contusion (R frontal) and frontal skull fracture

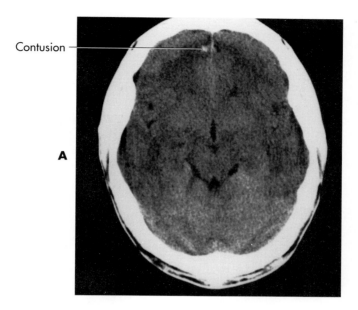

Contusion

FIGURE 2-25, A (Noncontrast)

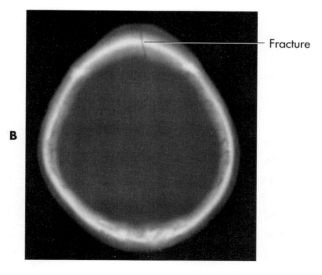

Fracture

FIGURE 2-25, B (Bone window)

Patient 2-26 • Focal hemorrhage

This patient was found unconscious with a possible but no definite history of trauma.

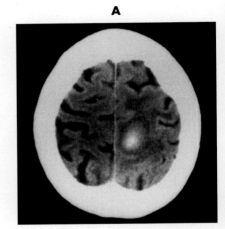

A

FIGURE 2-26, A (Noncontrast)

Focal area of hyperdensity indicating blood with a surrounding area of edema.

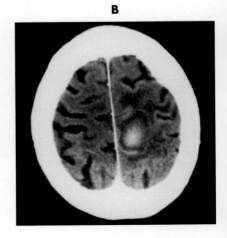

B

FIGURE 2-26, B (Contrast enhanced)

This is the same patient. Note that just around the ring of hypodensity indicating edema is a very thin white ring of hyperdensity. This is ring enhancement from contrast media (see Chapter 1). Contrast media was used to exclude an underlying neoplasm or AVM because the history for trauma was vague in this elderly patient. This is the expected finding of a resolving hematoma.

Noteworthy Point: Differential diagnosis of ring enhancing lesion: tumor, abscess, resolving hematoma.

Mixed SDH, Contusions, SAH, and Miscellaneous Injuries

Patient 2-27 • **Focal hemorrhagic contusions, acute subdural hematoma, and subarachnoid hemorrhage**

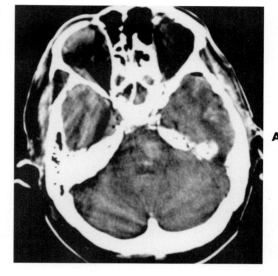

A

FIGURE 2-27, A (Noncontrast)

Focal hemorrhagic contusion within the brainstem (diffuse axonal injury) and obliteration of the ambient cisterns. Subcortical hemorrhagic contusion in the middle cranial fossa on the left. Artifact in the middle cranial fossa on the right.

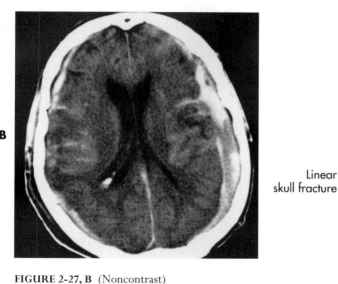

B

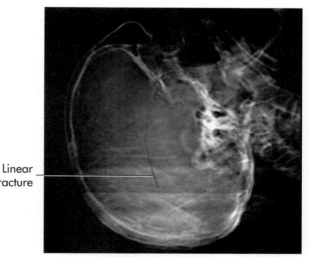

Linear skull fracture

C

FIGURE 2-27, B (Noncontrast)

Can you find the three abnormalities?

1. A large left temporal parietal acute subdural hematoma with clotted plus unclotted blood
2. A small right-sided subdural hematoma seen in the frontal and parietal regions
3. Subarachnoid blood within the cortical sulci

FIGURE 2-27, C (Noncontrast)

Patient 2-28 • Acute SDH and diffuse cerebral edema (L frontoparietal)

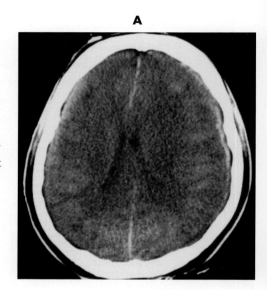

A

FIGURE 2-28, A (Noncontrast)

There is a thin hyperdense rim on the left side indicating a small acute subdural hematoma. Diffuse effacement of cortical sulci indicates diffuse cerebral edema.

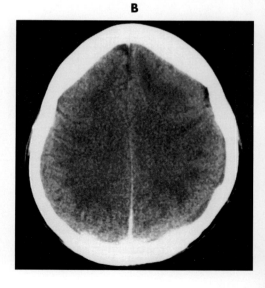

B

FIGURE 2-28, B (Noncontrast)

Two weeks later, the small isodense subdural hematoma on the left is invisible. The only clue to its presence is the effacement of the sulci of the left cerebral hemisphere compared to the other side. It is worth studying this image very carefully to appreciate the lack of the sulci on the left. Contrast enhancement may have confirmed the diagnosis; however, the patient also had an MRI scan, Figure 2-28, C.

Noteworthy Point: When reading CT scans, one must always ask the question, "Do the sulci extend out to the inner table on both sides?" Considering this question, you will appreciate the abnormality in Figure 2-28, *B*, and realize that further imaging is necessary.

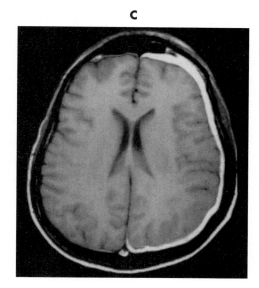

FIGURE 2-28, C (MRI noncontrast)

The sulcal effacement in Figure 2-28, B, required further investigation. The MRI shows a thin subacute subdural hematoma enclosing the entire left hemisphere. This appears bright on this T1W image because of paramagnetic effects of extracellular methemoglobin.

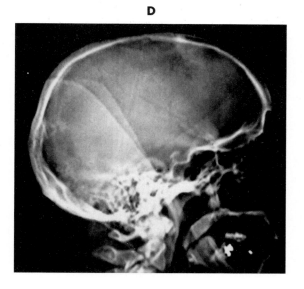

FIGURE 2-28, D (Scout view)

In keeping with the forces needed to cause an acute SDH this patient also suffered a fracture of C2 of the hangman's variety. This serves as a reminder to read all parts of all images.

Patient 2-29 • **Depressed skull fracture, parietal contusion, basal skull fracture through mastoid air cells, air in scalp hematoma (L)**

A

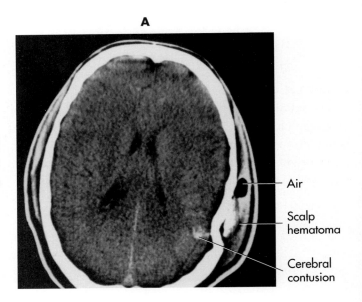

FIGURE 2-29, A (Noncontrast)

The air in the scalp hematoma could be from a scalp laceration or have tracked from the mastoid air cells through the fracture into the scalp hematoma.

Air

Scalp hematoma

Cerebral contusion

B

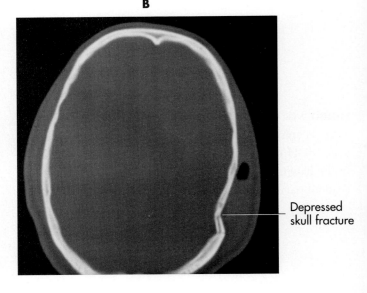

FIGURE 2-29, B (Bone window)

Depressed skull fracture

C

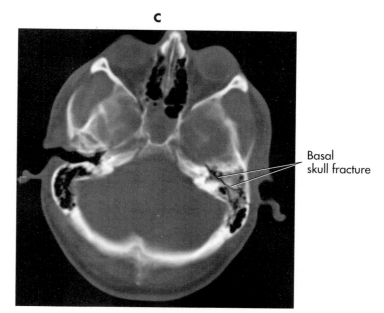

FIGURE 2-29, C (Bone window)

Basal
skull fracture

D

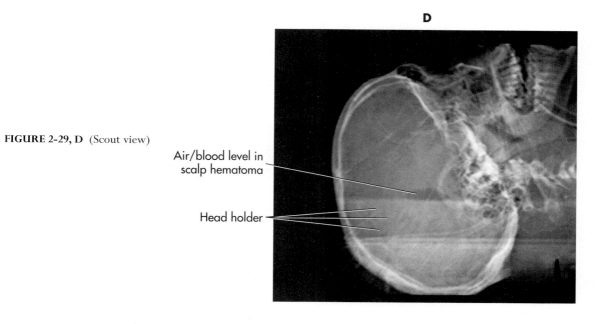

FIGURE 2-29, D (Scout view)

Air/blood level in
scalp hematoma

Head holder

Patient 2-30 • Acute SDH at tentorium (R), frontal contusion (L), traumatic SAH (R Sylvian fissure)

FIGURE 2-30 (Noncontrast)

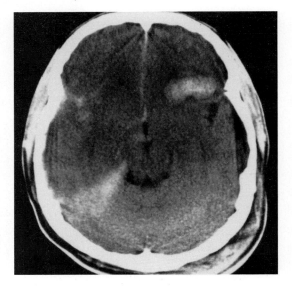

Patient 2-31 • Acute SDH (R) with evolution of contusion

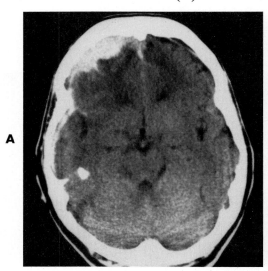

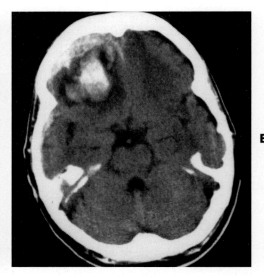

A

B

FIGURE 2-31, A (Noncontrast)
Acute SDH (R frontal) on day 1.

FIGURE 2-31, B (Noncontrast)
Five days later, the hemorrhagic contusion that was not apparent on day 1 is seen and this is the main cause of the patient's morbidity.

CHAPTER 3

ISCHEMIC STROKE

CT has revolutionized the assessment of patients who present with an acute neurologic deficit. A plain CT scan performed in the emergency setting can quickly exclude the presence of intracranial hemorrhage or space occupying lesion as the cause of the acute neurologic dysfunction.

Having excluded other causes for the neurologic dysfunction, a patient with a persistent neurologic deficit of only a few hours duration may have an entirely normal CT scan. This is not inconsistent with the diagnosis of cerebral infarction. These infarctions can be secondary to embolic phenomenon or, less likely, thrombosis of major supply arteries. Cells deprived of blood flow and therefore oxygenation rapidly progress from ischemia to actual infarction, particularly centrally, and are usually irreversibly damaged unless reperfusion is quickly reestablished. The cells in the more peripheral area of ischemia, often known as the "penumbra," may remain viable in an ischemic state for many hours. Ischemia produces energy depletion in the affected cells and loss of ion homeostasis. The resulting osmotically obligated water entry into the cell and anaerobic glucolysis causes intra and extra cellular metabolic acidosis. These cellular events associated with ischemia can become macroscopically detectable on CT scans within the first four to six hours. The changes that suggest acute infarction on plain CT scan are most often visualized in the middle cerebral artery territory and, when present, include:

1. The presence of a *hyperdense middle* or *anterior cerebral artery* due to the presence of the acute intraluminal thrombus.
2. *Mass effect*—slight effacement of adjacent ventricles, subarachnoid spaces, and sulci.
3. *Loss of the gray-white interface.* The normal contrast between white and gray matter is lost due to hypodense change in the gray matter, which is more sensitive to ischemia. This finding is seen earliest in the area of the insular cortex and later in the basal ganglia and cerebral cortex.

From 12 to 24 hours after the ictus, indistinct areas of low density may become apparent in the appropriate vascular distribution; this area becomes more conspicuous and circumscribed after 24 hours and there is increasing mass effect at this time that usually peaks between three to five days. Mass effect begins to decrease after five days and is usually resolved within two to four weeks. Between the second and third week in some 50% of cases, the infarct changes from low density to an isodense appearance before reverting to a more profound hypodense appearance. This has been termed CT "fogging" and may result from hyperemia after reperfusion, petechial hemorrhages, or macrophage activity. From approximately four weeks onward, the involved area becomes increasingly hypodense and is often associated with compensatory (ex vacuo) enlargement of the adjacent surrounding subarachnoid spaces and ventricles; at this point in time, the term encephalomalacia is used.

Hemorrhagic Infarct

When hemorrhagic transformation of an infarct occurs, it becomes apparent on CT four to ten days after the ictus. The hemorrhage appears as an area of hyperdensity and it is often located at the periphery of the central ischemic area.

Luxury Perfusion

In the month or so after an ischemic stroke, the contrast enhanced CT scan may be confusing unless one understands the findings associated with the term, luxury perfusion. This is relevant to emergency care because patients may be discharged from hospital after an acute stroke and re-present after sustaining new head trauma or have new neurologic symptoms.

Typically, from six days to six weeks after an acute ischemic stroke, abnormal contrast enhancement with CT imaging can often be seen in the area of infarction. The appearance demonstrates a gyral pattern in the cortex and homogeneous enhancement in the gray matter containing portions of the basal ganglia if they are infarcted as well. This appearance is secondary to leakage of contrast across a defective blood-brain barrier. The term luxury perfusion is commonly used to describe the above findings; however, it would probably be described more accurately as "hyperperfusion." Luxury perfusion is more correctly used to describe the increased circulation through an area of infarcted brain demonstrated angiographically by early venous drainage and transient angiographic blush.

Watershed Infarctions

Watershed infarctions are not due to embolic or thrombotic phenomenon. They are primarily the result of inadequate arterial perfusion. They are termed *watershed* because they occur in portions of the brain supplied by the most distal arterial branches of the major cerebral artery territories. The two cerebral watershed areas are located between: (1) the anterior and middle cerebral arteries and (2) between the middle and posterior cerebral arteries.

In most people, these areas invariably have an extremely tenuous blood supply. The decrease in arterial blood flow in the ipsilateral internal carotid artery can produce ischemia and/or infarction in the ipsilateral brain parenchyma within these watersheds. Typically, these infarctions are relatively confluent in nature and lack the CT feature of focal infarcts often seen after embolic phenomenon.

If there is systemic hypotension, hypoxemia, or cardiac arrest, these watershed type infarctions can be bilateral in nature.

Watershed infarctions of a unilateral distribution require further investigation to exclude stenosis or occlusion of the ipsilateral internal carotid artery. Bilateral watershed type infarctions suggest that a previous hypoxic, anoxic hypoperfusion, or cardiac arrest situation may have existed.

Ischemic Stroke

Patient 3-1 • **Hyperdense Middle Cerebral Artery (MCA) sign (L)**
• **Loss of Insular Stripe (L)**
• **MCA Territory Infarct (L)**

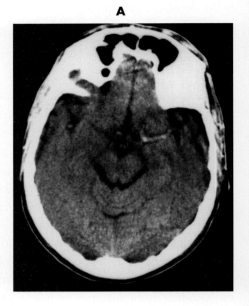

FIGURE 3-1, A (Noncontrast) Day 1

The horizontal linear hyperdensity on the left is due to a clot in the middle cerebral artery—the hyperdense MCA sign. Examination of the cerebral cortex here and in Figure 3-1, *B*, reveals no hypodensity in the MCA territory at this time to indicate infarction of the brain. There is no edema and no bleeding. The only indication of stroke on this image is the hyperdense MCA sign.

Noteworthy Point: The hyperdense MCA sign, when present, is the earliest abnormality seen on the CT scan with an acute infarction and represents a clot within the artery. In the majority of acute infarctions this sign is not present; however, it is specific and therefore an important CT finding. The diagnosis of the hyperdense MCA sign is made when this vessel appears to be more dense than other arteries of the same size in a *noncontrast* study and the patient has clinical findings of a severe MCA stroke. It is most often seen within the horizontal part of the middle cerebral artery. A false positive CT diagnosis of this sign could be made if the CT cut is through a large normal artery, which would appear mildly hyperdense compared to the surrounding tissue. However, in the case of a false positive, the patient would not have the expected dense hemiplegia. Fortunately, in most cases, the hyperdense vessel is indeed very hyperdense and there is no question of the diagnosis when correlated with the clinical findings.

B

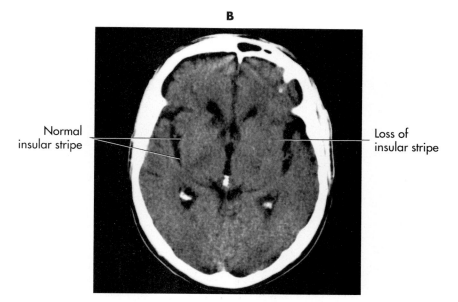

Normal insular stripe

Loss of insular stripe

FIGURE 3-1, B (Noncontrast) Day 1

Loss of the insular stripe is one of the more subtle but important indications of MCA stroke. First, look at the normal insula on the right. This is the cerebral cortex immediately medial to the Sylvian fissure. Normally this cortex appears as a thin white line, the so-called insular stripe. This is seen on the right side, which is normal. It is absent on the left-hand side due to ischemic stroke and represents early infarction of the gray matter of the insula.

continued

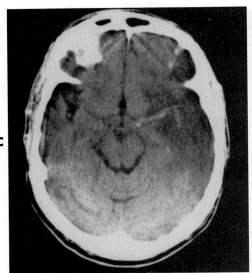

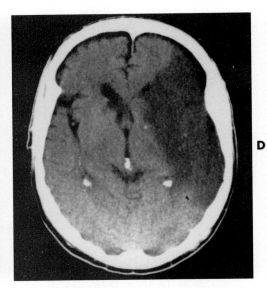

C

D

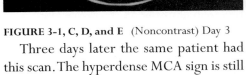

FIGURE 3-1, C, D, and E (Noncontrast) Day 3

Three days later the same patient had this scan. The hyperdense MCA sign is still present on 3-1, *C*, (this patient is from the prethrombolytic era). There is massive infarction of the brain in the left middle cerebral artery territory as evidenced by the hypodense area in 3-1, *C*, *D*, and *E*. There has been no hemorrhage and there is no significant midline shift.

E

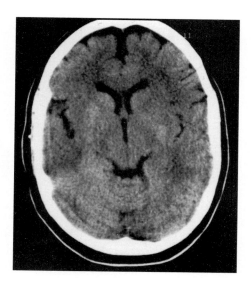

F

FIGURE 3-1, F (Noncontrast)

There is hypodensity in the outermost region of the cortex on the left side representing the MCA territory. The cortex just adjacent to the falx is normal, since it is supplied by the anterior cerebral artery (ACA) (see Figure 1-7, and Figures 3-7, *B*, and 3-8, *D*, for ACA infarct).

Patient 3-2 • Subtle MCA Territory Infarct (L)

FIGURE 3-2 (Noncontrast)

Look at the normal lentiform nucleus (putamen and globus pallidus) on the right side. Normally, this structure appears slightly hyperdense compared to the surrounding white matter because the lentiform nucleus is gray matter and it is bordered medially by the internal capsule and laterally by the external capsule, which are white matter. Now look at the abnormal lentiform nucleus on the left-hand side. There is the appearance of homogeneous hypodensity and this is due to early infarction of that structure, which falls within the MCA supply territory. A CT scan taken several days later confirmed a large MCA infarction. The insular stripe on the left is absent.

Patient 3-3 • Subtle MCA Infarct (R)

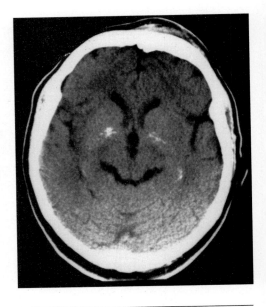

FIGURE 3-3 (Noncontrast)

The eye is easily distracted by the physiologic calcification in both basal ganglia, which is a common normal variant. The abnormal finding is the loss of the insular stripe on the right as explained in Figures 3-1 and 3-2.

Patient 3-4 • MCA Territory Infarction (L)

This scan was taken shortly after the onset of the patient's symptoms. We know this will be a large infarction because of the extent of the hypodensities that are present at this early stage.

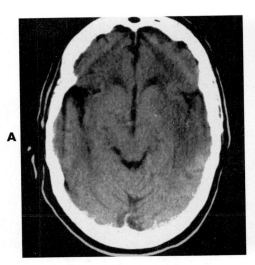
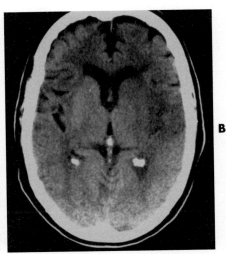

A

B

FIGURE 3-4 (Noncontrast)

A, On the left-hand side the following structures are hypodense due to infarction: (1) the basal ganglia, (2) insula (loss of insular stripe), and (3) temporal lobe. **B,** This is the next higher cut and shows the same findings in the left caudate and lentiform nuclei and frontal lobe.

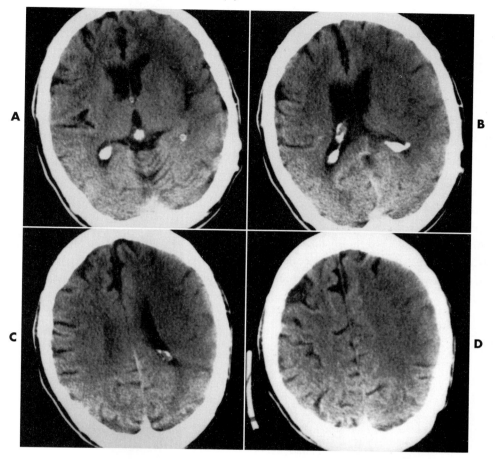

FIGURE 3-5, A-D (Noncontrast)

A, The insular stripe on the right-hand side is well seen but is absent on the left-hand side. There is also low density change in the frontal lobe due to infarction. **B**, The following signs of infarction are present:

1. There is loss of the gray-white differentiation in the left frontal lobe as compared to the right-hand side (i.e., the entire left frontal lobe appears hypodense compared to the other side). Careful study of this image is encouraged to appreciate this important diagnostic finding.

2. There is loss of the sulci when one examines the junction of the cortex and inner table of

the skull on the left-hand side compared to the right-hand side and this indicates local mass effect. There is also compression of the left lateral ventricle from the edema.

C, Again, it should be evident at first glance that the sulci of the left frontoparietal cortex are effaced. There is homogeneous hypodensity and loss of the gray-white differentiation due to infarction, edema, and local mass effect. **D**, Effacement of sulci and loss of gray-white differentiation of the left frontoparietal cortex. Note that the cortex just beside the falx on the left is normal, since this area is supplied by the anterior cerebral artery (ACA).

Patient 3-6 • Luxury Perfusion of MCA Infarct (R)

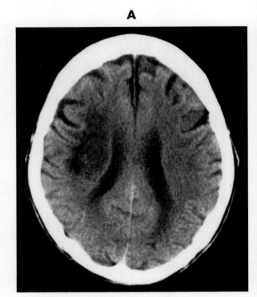

A

FIGURE 3-6, A (Noncontrast)

The hypodense area in the right frontal region represents an infarction in the right MCA territory. At a certain stage in the evolution of CT findings in infarction, the cortex can appear to be normal on a noncontrast CT, as seen in this case, even though the white matter is infarcted. Therefore this CT appears to have a subcortical abnormality without a cortical component and could be mistaken for edema associated with a neoplastic or inflammatory condition. The contrast enhanced scan on the same day, Figure 3-6, B, clarifies the diagnosis.

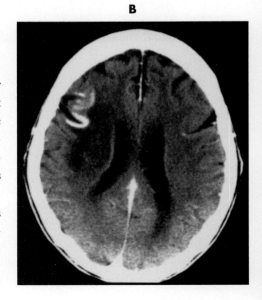

B

FIGURE 3-6, B (Contrast enhanced)

The contrast infused study shows gyriform enhancement. This is in keeping with luxury perfusion (see Chapter 3, p. 60), which represents leakage of intravascular contrast across a disrupted blood-brain barrier and confirms the presence of an accompanying cortical infarct. Luxury perfusion involves only gray matter, either cortex or basal ganglia, and is a finding that may be present one to six weeks postinfarction.

The hyperdense structure in the posterior midline is a normal finding with contrast enhancement: the straight sinus and vein of Galen (see Figures 1-10, *E*, and 9-1 to 9-3).

Patient 3-7 • Anterior Cerebral Artery Territory Infarct (L)

Anterior cerebral artery (ACA) strokes are less common than MCA infarcts. There may be a tendency to overlook the CT findings because they are located on the higher cuts and the abnormalities are toward the midline rather than the convexity as seen with other territory infarcts.

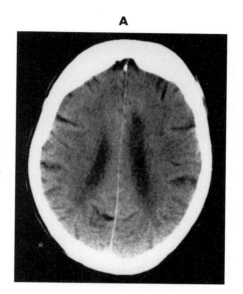

A

FIGURE 3-7, A (Noncontrast)

The left lateral ventricle is more prominent than the right side. This could be a variation of normal but there is such a great discrepancy between the two sides that careful examination is required of that region in the adjacent cuts.

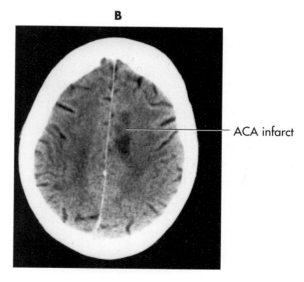

B

ACA infarct

FIGURE 3-7, B (Noncontrast)

Hypodensity of the medial cortex just to the left of the falx is due to ACA territory infarct (see Chapter 1, Figure 1-7).

Patient 3-8 • Infarction in the ACA and MCA Territories (L)
• Hyperdense Vessel Signs

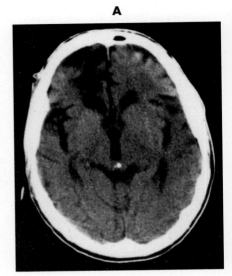

A

FIGURE 3-8, A (Noncontrast) Day 1

The patient had this initial CT scan that shows an old infarct in the right frontal lobe and some atrophy as evidenced by prominent Sylvian fissures and anterior interhemispheric fissure and dilated third ventricle. The same patient had a CT scan two days later (Figure 3-8, *B*) after developing a decreased level of consciousness and a dense right hemiparesis.

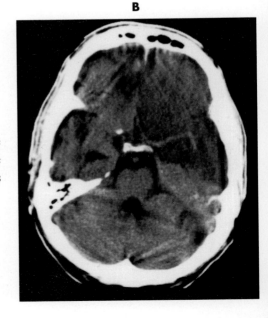

B

FIGURE 3-8, B (Noncontrast) Day 3

The hyperdense vessel sign is present in the left middle cerebral artery and the left anterior cerebral artery. There are low density changes in the corresponding territories due to infarction.

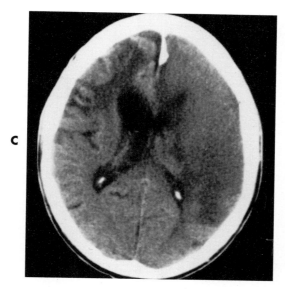

FIGURE 3-8, C (Noncontrast)

There is marked hypodensity in the left MCA territory. The Sylvian fissure is completely obliterated as compared to the other side. The left lateral ventricle is compressed from edema. Note how the occipital lobe, which is supplied by the posterior cerebral artery, is intact on the left side. There is incidental note of calcification within the falx anteriorly. The hypodense area in the right frontal lobe corresponds to the old right frontal infarct.

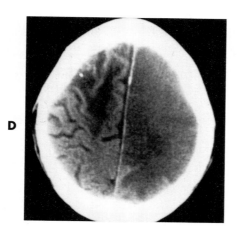

FIGURE 3-8, D (Noncontrast)

The entire left hemisphere appears infarcted. Remember that the anterior cerebral artery supplies the medial part of the brain just adjacent to the falx.

It may be useful to return to Figure 3-1, *F*, (isolated MCA infarct) to compare it with this CT scan of infarcts of both the MCA and ACA territories.

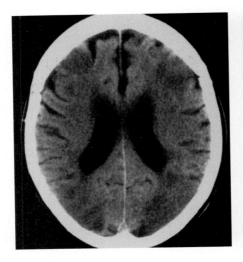
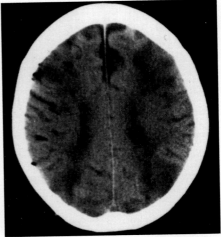
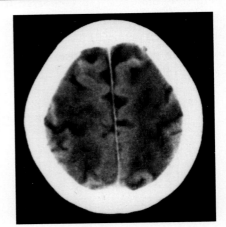

FIGURE 3-9 (Noncontrast)

The hypodensities in left and right frontal and parietal regions are due to global hypoperfusion or hypoxemia and represent infarctions in the watershed zone between the ACA and MCA. See p. 65 for explanation of watershed infarction.

Patient 3-10 • Occipital Lobe Infarct (L)

We are reminded that this is the occipital lobe and not the posterior fossa because at this level we are above the internal occipital protuberance and tentorial incisura. If there is any question, one can orient the level of the slice with the scout views (see Figure 1-8, *A*). The occipital lobes are supplied by the terminal branches of the posterior cerebral artery.

A

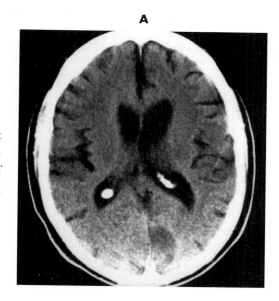

FIGURE 3-10, A (Noncontrast)

There is a well circumscribed hypodensity in the left occipital lobe. This is somewhat obscured by streak artifact from the internal occipital protuberance. Also of note are the prominent lateral ventricles and cortical sulci in keeping with age related atrophy.

B

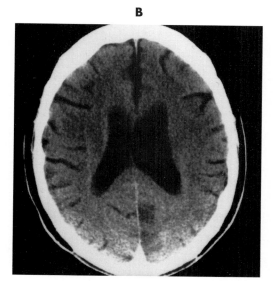

FIGURE 3-10, B (Noncontrast)

Persistence of the abnormality on two cuts confirms the occipital infarct.

Patient 3-11 • Occipital Lobe Infarct (Posterior Cerebral Artery Territory) (R)

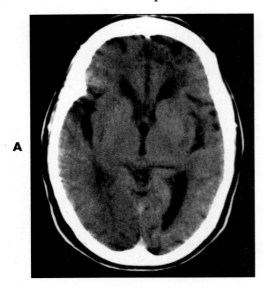

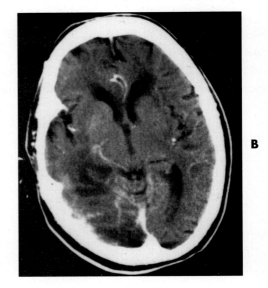

FIGURE 3-11, A (Noncontrast) Day 1

The large right occipital hypodensity with mass effect (sulci effaced) is due to infarction.

FIGURE 3-11, B (Contrast enhanced) Day 8

One week later the patchy contrast enhanced area within the hypodensity probably indicates early luxury perfusion.

Patient 3-12 • Basilar Artery Territory Infarction

The territory of the left and right posterior cerebral arteries are infarcted and this includes the brainstem, right cerebellum, both occipital lobes, posterior portion of both temporal lobes, and left thalamus. To infarct both sides, the artery proximal to the posterior cerebral arteries must be involved and this is the basilar artery. Basilar artery infarcts have a poor prognosis.

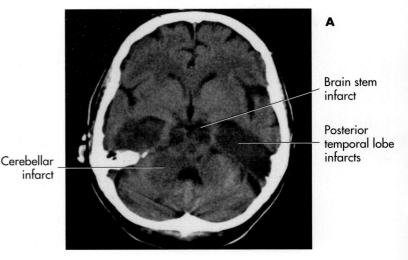

Brain stem infarct

Posterior temporal lobe infarcts

Cerebellar infarct

FIGURE 3-12, A (Noncontrast)

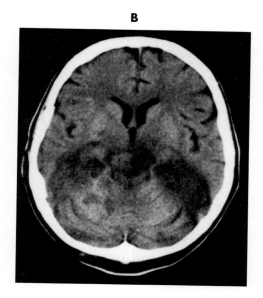

FIGURE 3-12, B (Noncontrast)

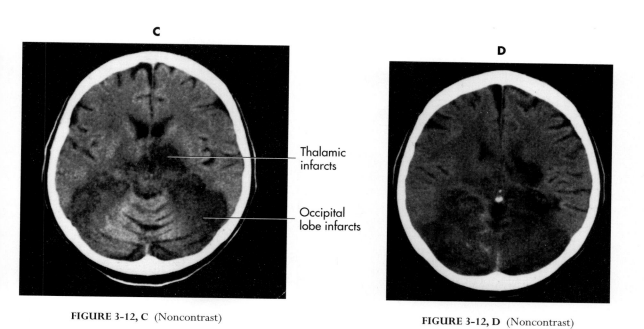

FIGURE 3-12, C (Noncontrast)

Thalamic infarcts

Occipital lobe infarcts

FIGURE 3-12, D (Noncontrast)

Patient 3-13 • Infarction Cerebellar Hemisphere (R)

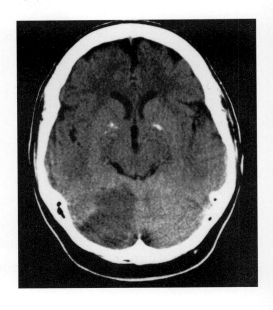

FIGURE 3-13 (Noncontrast)

Note that this is the cerebellum, not the occipital lobe. The calcification of both basal ganglia is an incidental finding.

Patient 3-14 • Brainstem Infarction

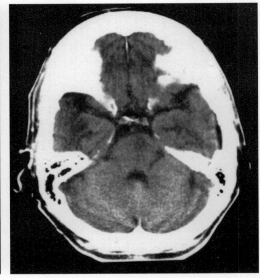

A

B

Brainstem
infarct

FIGURE 3-14, A (Noncontrast) Day 1

FIGURE 3-14, B (Noncontrast) Day 1

An unlabelled version of the same image in A better demonstrates the subtle abnormality.

FIGURE 3-14, C (Noncontrast) Day 4

Three days later, the infarct is more readily apparent.

Patient 3-15 • Venous Thrombosis (Superior Sagittal Sinus and Vein of Galen)

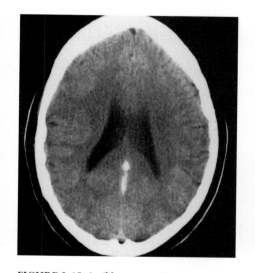

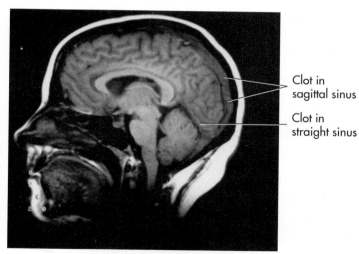

Clot in
sagittal sinus

Clot in
straight sinus

FIGURE 3-15, A (Noncontrast)

The vein of Galen and straight sinus appear hyperdense and thickened due to thrombosis on this noncontrast study. (The variants of normal of these structures on noncontrast CT, Figures 9-1 to 9-3, are not as dense or as thick as seen in this case.)

FIGURE 3-15, B (Noncontrast MRI)

On this noncontrast T1W sagittal MRI the thrombosed sagittal sinus is seen as an abnormally thickened structure.

Patient 3-16 • Sagittal Sinus Thrombosis (Delta Sign)

This patient complained of severe, sudden headache that was much worse when recumbent than sitting.

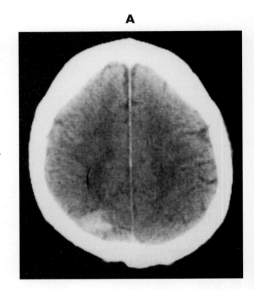

A

FIGURE 3-16, A (Noncontrast)

There is a hemorrhagic lesion of the right posterior parietal cortex of undetermined etiology.

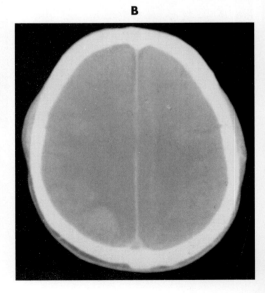

B

FIGURE 3-16, B (Contrast Enhanced)

Normally with contrast the blood within the sagittal sinus should appear hyperdense (see Figure 1-10, *E* and Figure 6-6, *C*). A triangular hypodense area is present due to blood clot within the sinus. This is called the delta sign. Adjustment of the windows setting for this image was necessary to discriminate the density of the clot from that of the adjacent bone. Referring to Figure 3-16, *A*, this can now be interpreted as a hemorrhagic infarction of a venous nature, in keeping with the clinical course of sagittal sinus thrombosis.

Patient 3-17 • Venous Dural Sinus Thrombosis

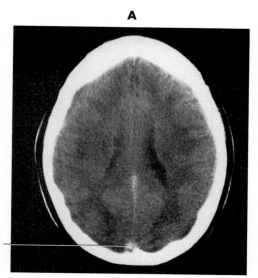

Thrombosed
sagittal sinus

FIGURE 3-17, A (Noncontrast)

The superior sagittal sinus is slightly prominent and slightly dense but could be within normal limits. However, the higher cut Figure 3-17, *B*, that shows the superior sagittal sinus in profile reveals that it is thickened and hyperdense. In the right clinical setting this should raise the possibility of superior sagittal sinus thrombosis. Further investigation (MRI or angiography) is required to confirm the diagnosis.

FIGURE 3-17, B (Noncontrast)

This cut through the upper brain should always be examined with the same diligence as the rest of the scan so as not to miss important findings as seen here. The vertical linear hyperdensity is clot within the superior sagittal sinus. See Figure 1-8 *L* for comparison to a normal noncontrast study at this level.

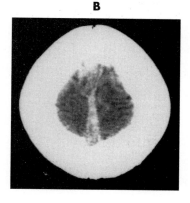

Patient 3-18 • Lacunar Infarction

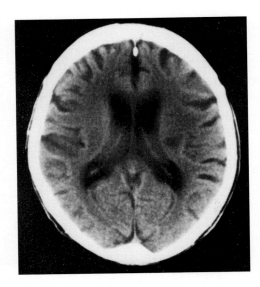

FIGURE 3-18 (Noncontrast)

Lacunar infarction in the left corona radiata. This results from occlusion of the small end vessels that supply the white matter and deep gray matter due to the effects of hypertension. The infarcted tissue becomes cystic, hence the name lacuna.

CHAPTER 4

SUBARACHNOID HEMORRHAGE AND ANEURYSMS

Severe or sudden headache is one of the more common reasons for patients to present to the emergency department and rupture of a berry aneurysm is a key diagnostic consideration. Approximately 3% of the population harbor an intracranial aneurysm and each intracranial aneurysm has approximately a 2% to 3% cumulative annual risk of rupture. Before complete rupture of an aneurysm with potentially devastating consequences, many patients will have an acute milder headache due to a sentinel hemorrhage. A ruptured aneurysm will bleed into the subarachnoid space and in some patients, into the cerebral parenchyma, ventricles, or subdural space.

It is crucial that the diagnosis of subarachnoid hemorrhage (SAH) be established because these patients require further neuroimaging and potential definitive treatment.

- *A nonenhanced CT scan is the quickest, most accurate, and most readily available noninvasive examination for the evaluation of acute headache.*
- It can accurately detect the presence of acute intracranial hemorrhage within minutes after acute clot retraction and can locate the hemorrhage in the intracerebral, subarachnoid, subdural, or epidural compartments.
- *In comparison to the CT scan, MRI scans are poor for detecting acute hemorrhage.*
- The CT scan can also distinguish between other common causes of acute headache, such as space occupying lesions or hydrocephalus.

Acute subarachnoid hemorrhage appears as a hyperdense collection (white), most commonly in the basal cisterns. This hyperdensity is visible within minutes of the onset of hemorrhage and decreases steadily until it becomes isodense to CSF within one week. Therefore the CT becomes less sensitive in determining SAH as the time from onset of headache passes.

Accompanying the acute subarachnoid hemorrhage may be evidence of acute intraventricular, intraparenchymal and subdural hemorrhage, and hydrocephalus. The hydrocephalus may be obstructive in nature (noncommunicating) due to plugging of the cerebral aqueduct, or nonobstructive (communicating) due to plugging of the arachnoid granulations, which results in decreased uptake of CSF. *The earliest sign of this hydrocephalus is often dilation of the temporal horns,* and the size of these structures must always be evaluated when reading a CT.

A normal CT scan is reassuring but does not absolutely exclude the presence of a subarachnoid hemorrhage if the hemorrhage is extremely small, has occurred several days previously, or was located low in the posterior fossa or in the spinal axis. In patients in whom there is a high clinical suspicion that the headache resulted from subarachnoid hemorrhage, a lumbar puncture would be the next examination of choice, looking for small quantities of red blood cells in the CSF and/or xanthochromia.

Other causes of SAH are bleeding from an arteriovenous malformation (AVM), trauma, hemorrhagic tumor, and dural malformation. The images that follow illustrate the findings of SAH, which may be quite subtle in sentinel bleeds.

CT Interpretation in SAH

> **Practical Points**
> Scrutinize the following areas of the CT systematically for the presence of sub-arachnoid blood:
> the basal cisterns
> the Sylvian fissures
> the interhemispheric fissure.
> Dilation of the temporal horns is a sign of hydrocephalus, which may indicate the possibility of SAH.

Subarachnoid Hemorrhage

Patient 4-1

Noteworthy Point: The so-called "star sign" refers to blood radiating like points of a star from the basal cisterns and often into the interhemispheric fissure.

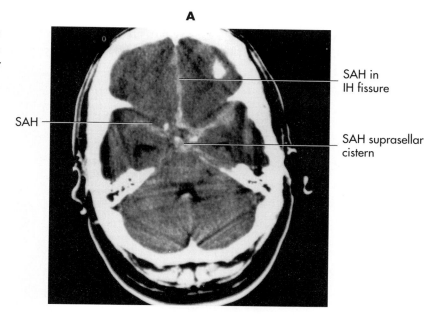

SAH in IH fissure

SAH

SAH suprasellar cistern

FIGURE 4-1, A (Noncontrast)

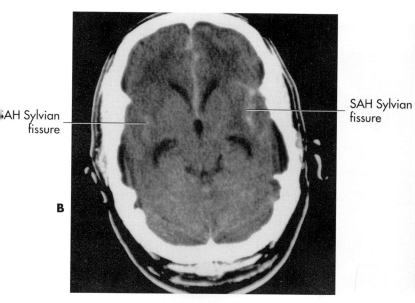

SAH Sylvian fissure

SAH Sylvian fissure

FIGURE 4-1, B (Noncontrast)

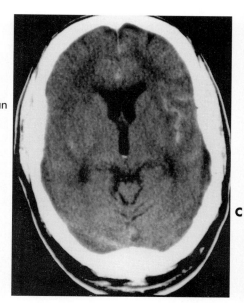

FIGURE 4-1, C (Noncontrast)

Acute hemorrhage in the left Sylvian fissure and in the left frontal sulcus. Streak artifact from the internal occipital protuberance is present.

Patient 4-2 • Classic Subarachnoid Hemorrhage

Noteworthy Point: Whenever there is nontraumatic subarachnoid hemorrhage or intraventricular hemorrhage without an underlying intracerebral hemorrhage, an aneurysm or AVM must be excluded by further investigations.

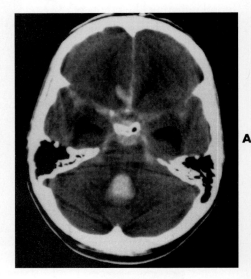

FIGURE 4-2, A (Noncontrast)

The star sign is seen (see Figure 4-1, *A*). There is hemorrhage in the fourth ventricle. The temporal horns are markedly dilated.

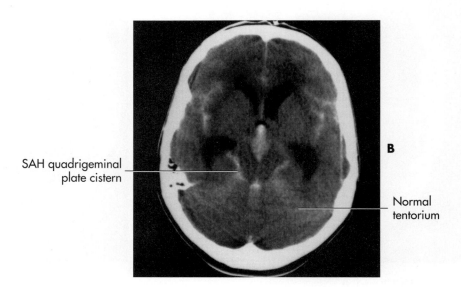

SAH quadrigeminal plate cistern

Normal tentorium

FIGURE 4-2, B (Noncontrast)

Acute hemorrhage in both Sylvian fissures, the quadrigeminal plate cistern, and the third ventricle. Marked dilatation of the temporal horns due to hydrocephalus is present.

C

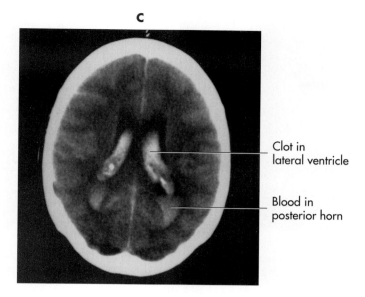

Clot in
lateral ventricle

Blood in
posterior horn

FIGURE 4-2, C (Noncontrast)

Patient 4-3 • Subarachnoid Hemorrhage

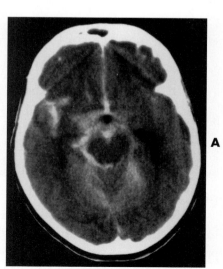

A

FIGURE 4-3, A (Noncontrast)

Acute hemorrhage in the following cisterns and subarachnoid spaces: right Sylvian fissure, the suprasellar cistern, the ambient and quadrigeminal plate cisterns. The interhemispheric fissure appears quite hyperdense and this is due to hemorrhage in the fissure on either side of the falx. The temporal horns are dilated. There is some hazy hyperdensity in the region of the tentorium that represents hemorrhage in the superior cerebellar cisterns and this is better seen on the next higher cut (Figure 4-3, *B*).

Continued

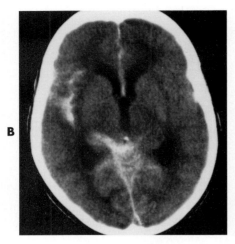

FIGURE 4-3, B (Noncontrast)

Subarachnoid blood in the right Sylvian fissure, interhemispheric fissure, and the superior cerebellar cisterns.

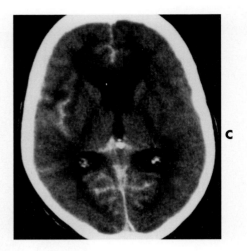

FIGURE 4-3, C (Noncontrast)

Acute hemorrhage in the sulci of the occipital lobe, right Sylvian, and anterior interhemispheric fissures.

Patient 4-4 • Subarachnoid Hemorrhage

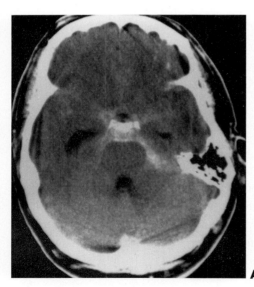

SAH interpedunucular cistern

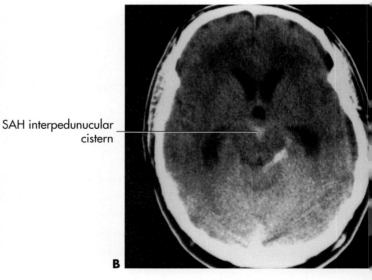

FIGURE 4-4, A (Noncontrast)

The star sign is present due to SAH in the basal cisterns, although more subtle than in previous examples. The dilatation of the temporal horns is a clue to look carefully for SAH.

FIGURE 4-4, B (Noncontrast)

SAH in the interpeduncular cistern and the left side of the ambient cistern. The temporal horns and third ventricle are markedly dilated.

Patient 4-5 • Acute SAH

This patient is somewhat atypical in that there is no hydrocephalus present at this stage, which is usually expected with this degree of hemorrhage.

FIGURE 4-5, A (Noncontrast)

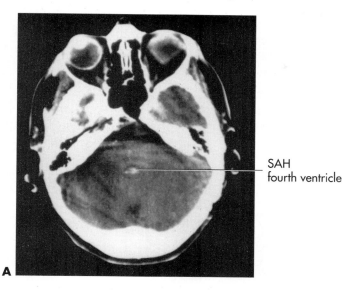

SAH
fourth ventricle

A

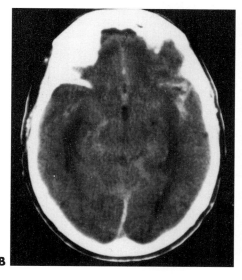

B

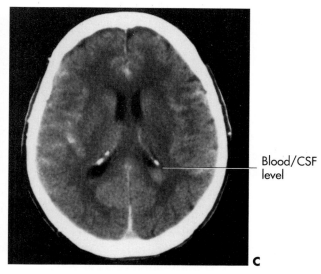

Blood/CSF
level

C

FIGURE 4-5, B (Noncontrast)

Hemorrhage in the left Sylvian fissure, the right side of the ambient cistern, and a faint suggestion of hemorrhage in the right Sylvian fissure.

FIGURE 4-5, C (Noncontrast)

Subarachnoid hemorrhage is present in the sulci of both frontal lobes and the anterior interhemispheric fissure. There is a CSF/blood level in both posterior horns, more prominent on the left.

Patient 4-6 • **Acute SAH**

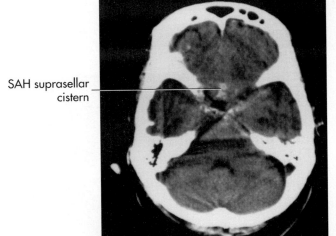

SAH suprasellar
cistern

A

FIGURE 4-6, A (Noncontrast)

There is blood in the suprasellar cistern. This should not be mistaken for streak artifact from the adjacent bony ridges.

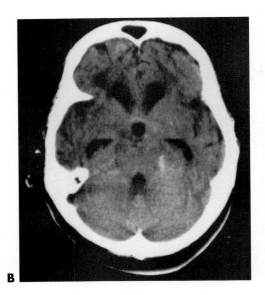

B

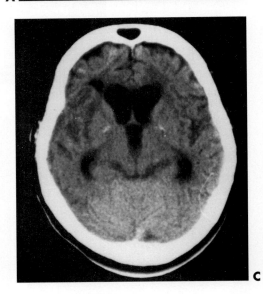

C

FIGURE 4-6, B (Noncontrast)

There is blood in the left ambient cistern that should not be mistakenly interpreted as an asymmetric cut through the petrous temporal bone. The temporal horns are dilated, as is the third ventricle, due to hydrocephalus.

FIGURE 4-6, C (Noncontrast)

The only abnormality on this image compatible with SAH is hydrocephalus. The tiny hyperdense areas in the left and right basal ganglia represent calcification in the basal ganglia, which is a commonly observed normal finding on CT scans. This should not be mistaken for hemorrhage in this area. Also there is a subcortical hypodensity in the right frontal lobe that is consistent with an old infarction.

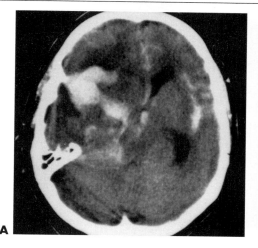 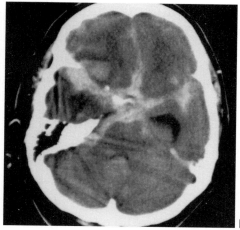

FIGURE 4-7 (Noncontrast)

A, Star sign. **B**, A large clot is seen in the right insula and basal ganglia and there is subarachnoid blood in the anterior interhemispheric fissure, the left and right Sylvian fissures, left frontal sulci, and the third ventricle. Note the subfalcial herniation to the left. There is marked dilatation of the left temporal horn.

Noteworthy Point: The nontraumatic SAH should be considered the primary insult regardless of whether or not there is intracerebral hemorrhage. Large clots like this in the frontotemporal region are frequently associated with middle cerebral artery (MCA) aneurysm.

Patient 4-8 • **SAH**

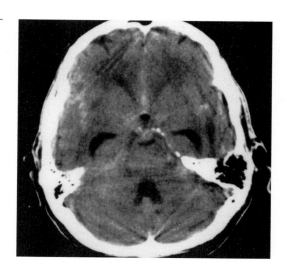

FIGURE 4-8 (Noncontrast)

Subtle star sign plus SAH in R Sylvian fissure and hydrocephalus.

Patient 4-9 • Intracranial Hemorrhage

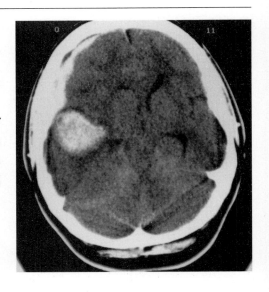

FIGURE 4-9 (Noncontrast)

A large intaparenchymal hemorrhage in the vicinity of the Sylvian fissure is commonly seen with ruptured middle cerebral artery aneurysms. Note the associated extension of hemorrhage into the right frontal subdural space causing an acute SDH and subfalcial herniation.

Patient 4-10 • SAH Due to Aneurysm of Right Middle Cerebral Artery

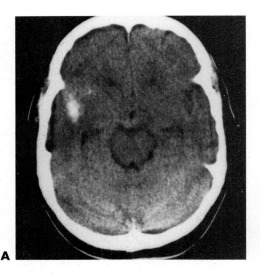

A

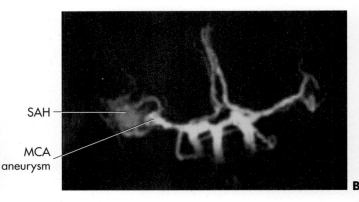

B

FIGURE 4-10, A (Noncontrast)

There is acute hemorrhage isolated to the right Sylvian fissure. Compare this to the normal, hypodense appearance of the subarachnoid space in the Sylvian fissure on the left side. The Sylvian fissure is a frequent location for subarachnoid hemorrhage.

FIGURE 4-10, B (MR angiogram)

This 3D time of flight magnetic resonance angiogram demonstrates the aneurysm of the middle cerebral artery and associated SAH.

Patient 4-11 • Normal CT

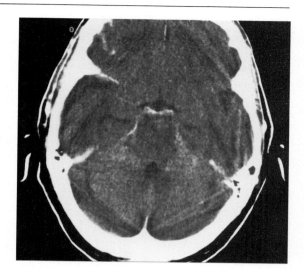

FIGURE 4-11 (Noncontrast)

This is a normal scan. The normal tentorial density should not be mistaken for acute SAH.

Patient 4-12 • Subtle SAH

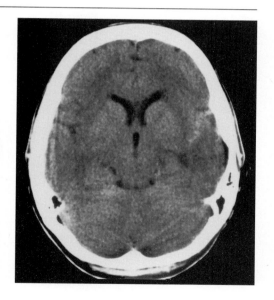

FIGURE 4-12 (Noncontrast)

The right Sylvian fissure is completely normal. Comparison with the other side reveals some hyperdensity within the left Sylvian fissure due to acute subarachnoid hemorrhage. Angiogram demonstrated a 5 mm aneurysm at the left MCA trifurcation.

Patient 4-13 • Subtle SAH

This patient presented with sudden onset of headache. There are subtle indications of subarachnoid hemorrhage.

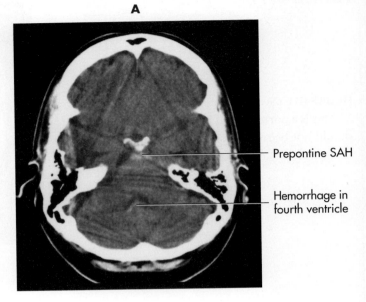

FIGURE 4-13, A (Noncontrast)

— Prepontine SAH

Hemorrhage in fourth ventricle

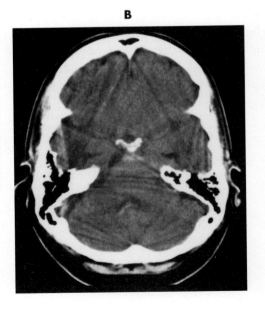

B

FIGURE 4-13, B (Noncontrast)

An unlabelled version of the same image in Figure 4-13, A, is provided to better appreciate the subtle abnormality.

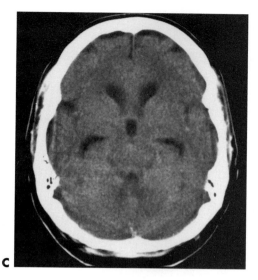

C

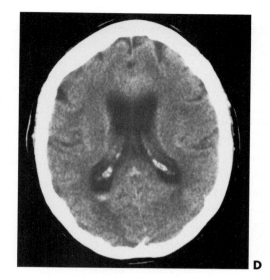

D

FIGURE 4-13, C (Noncontrast)

The temporal horns are dilated. This would mandate thorough investigation for aneurysm in this patient even if the pre-pontine blood in Figure 4-13, A, was not appreciated.

FIGURE 4-13, D (Noncontrast)

There is a straight horizontal line in the posterior horns of both lateral ventricles indicating blood/CSF fluid level. This is more subtle than that seen in Figures 4-2, C, and 4-5, C.

Patient 4-14 • Dilated Temporal Horns

FIGURE 4-14 (Noncontrast)

This patient had an excellent history for subarachnoid hemorrhage but no definite hemorrhage is seen on the CT scans. However, this is definitely an abnormal CT scan due to the marked dilatation of the temporal horns in keeping with mild hydrocephalus. Angiography in this patient showed a left posterior communicating artery aneurysm.

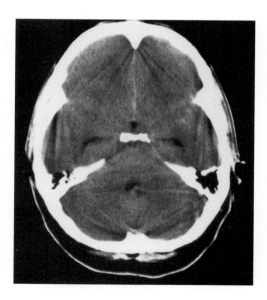

Patient 4-15 • Aneurysm MCA (R) (Contrast Enhanced)

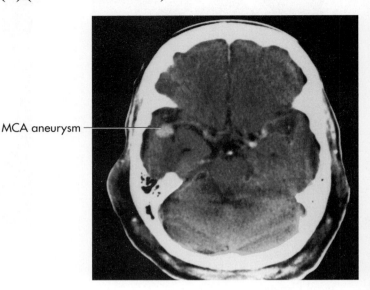

FIGURE 4-15 (Contrast Enhanced)

This patient received a contrast enhanced CT scan as part of an investigation to rule out cerebral abscess associated with sepsis. The scan was normal in this regard but incidentally demonstrated a very large aneurysm of the right middle cerebral artery.

MCA aneurysm

Patient 4-16 • Fusiform Atherosclerotic Aneurysm of the Basilar Artery

FIGURE 4-16, A (Noncontrast)

Cursory examination of this CT scan may lead one to focus on the hyperdensity in the left frontal lobe. However, comparison with the cut below (which is not reproduced due to space) shows that this is an asymmetric cut through the normal orbital roof.

Systematic examination includes examination of the structures in the midline. There is a round, tubular hyperdensity just posterior to the sphenoid sinus that corresponds to the abnormality seen on Figure 4-16, *B*, which is a discrete hyperdensity in the region of the pons. The diagnosis is most likely a giant aneurysm of the basilar artery. The differential diagnosis includes an acute brainstem hemorrhage. The final diagnosis is evident on the MRI scan: a fusiform atherosclerotic aneurysm that usually results in brainstem infarction rather than SAH.

A

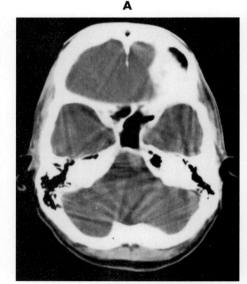

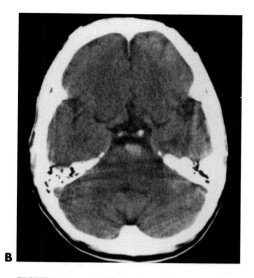

B

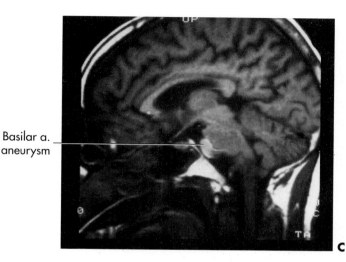

Basilar a.
aneurysm

C

FIGURE 4-16, B (Noncontrast)
Hyperdensity in pons.

FIGURE 4-16, C (MRI Noncontrast)

Patient 4-17 • Giant Aneurysm

FIGURE 4-17 (Noncontrast)

At first glance, the main striking feature is the prominence of the interhemispheric fissure secondary to cerebral atrophy. In the setting of this amount of atrophy, the dilatation of the temporal horns is probably due to the atrophy.

In the midline, there is a round, well-circumscribed abnormality located in the suprasellar cistern that has the same density as the adjacent brain. The differential diagnosis is a giant aneurysm versus a suprasellar tumor. Midline abnormalities on the CT scan are easy to miss versus abnormalities on one side of the brain (our eye picks this up easily because we make comparisons with the other side).

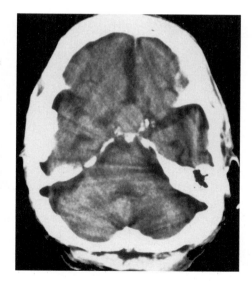

Patient 4-18 • Giant Aneurysm
(Contrast Enhanced)

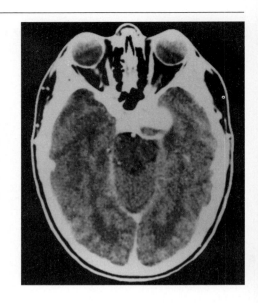

FIGURE 4-18 (Contrast Enhanced)

This patient presented with diplopia. This contrast-enhanced CT scan demonstrates a giant aneurysm in the region of the left cavernous sinus. The hypodense area represents clot within the aneurysm. Angiography demonstrated a giant aneurysm from the cavernous sinus portion of the left carotid artery.

Patient 4-19 • Giant Aneurysm

Giant aneurysm

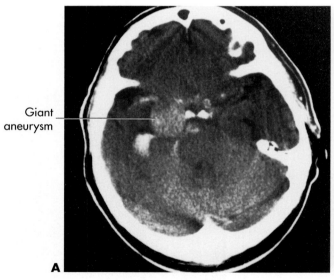

A

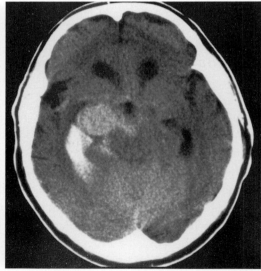

B

FIGURE 4-19, A (Noncontrast)

FIGURE 4-19, B (Noncontrast)

In the region of the right posterior communicating artery, there is a round well-defined hyperdense area representing a giant aneurysm. Both images from this patient demonstrate acute hemorrhage into the right temporal horn, as well as hemorrhage into the interpeduncular cistern.

Patient 4-20 • MCA Aneurysm (R)

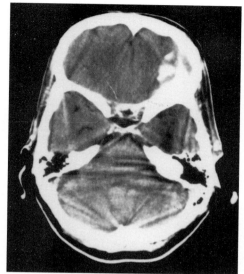

A

FIGURE 4-20, A (Noncontrast)

There is a discrete hypodensity in the middle cranial fossa on the right in the region of the MCA, which was further evaluated with contrast enhancement, Figure 4-20, *B*.

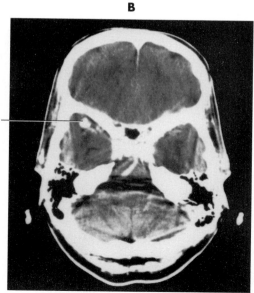

B

MCA
aneurysm

FIGURE 4-20, B (Contrast Enhanced)

Do not mistake the aneurysm, which is well seen with contrast enhancement, for bone.

CHAPTER 5

NONTRAUMATIC HEMORRHAGE AND VASCULAR MALFORMATIONS

Intracerebral hemorrhage, independent of its cause, is a common cause of acute neurologic dysfunction and therefore is a common finding on CT scans of the head performed in the emergency setting. The most common causes of nontraumatic hemorrhage are acute hypertension, cerebral aneurysms, and vascular malformations.

Hypertension

Hypertension is the most common cause of nontraumatic intracranial hemorrhage in adults. These are typically seen in elderly patients in association with systemic hypertension. In some cases ruptured microaneurysms of the deep perforating vessels, particularly the lateral lenticulostriate arteries, have been implicated. Hypertensive intracranial hemorrhage has a predilection for the areas supplied by the penetrating branches of the middle cerebral and basilar arteries. In decreasing order of frequency these involve the putamen and external capsule, thalamus, pons, cerebellum, and subcortical white matter. In approximately one half of these hypertensive hemorrhages there is dissection into the ventricular system. These acute intracerebral hemorrhages appear as focal areas of high density on plain CT examinations.

Aneurysms

Although intracranial aneurysms are most frequently associated with acute subarachnoid hemorrhage, they frequently have an associated intracerebral hemorrhage or "clot." This is most commonly seen in the temporal region with middle cerebral artery bifurcation aneurysms. Far less frequently and usually considerably smaller in size is the intracerebral hemorrhage that can be associated in the frontal regions with anterior communicating artery aneurysms. Because of the importance of aneurysms and their particular features on CT when they rupture they are discussed separately in the chapter on subarachnoid hemorrhage.

Vascular Malformations

There are four types of vascular malformations and only two (arteriovenous malformations and cavernous angioma) are frequently associated with intracranial hemorrhage.

Arteriovenous Malformation

Arteriovenous malformation (AVM) is the most common type of vascular abnormality. These lesions are congenital in nature, usually solitary, and consist of dilated arteries and veins without an intervening capillary bed. They frequently present between the ages of 20 and 40 years with acute hemorrhage in 50% and seizures in approximately 25%. They are associated with approximately a 2% to 3% per year cumulative risk of hemorrhage and produce a neurologic deficit at the time of hemorrhage in approximately 25% of patients.

AVMs unassociated with acute intracerebral hemorrhage may appear on a plain CT scan as subtle areas of increased density, often with a serpiginous-type shape. There may be associated calcification and there is usually subtle mass effect. These lesions enhance intensely with contrast, producing "a bag of worms" appearance.

Cavernous Angioma

A far less frequent cause of intracranial hemorrhage is a cavernous angioma. Patients with these lesions are estimated to have symptomatic intracranial hemorrhages at a rate of approximately 0.5% to 1% per year. Occult bleeds without clinical manifestations, however, are more common. These lesions consist of a lobulated collection of dilated endothelial lined spaces. There is no normal intervening brain within the lesion. The lesion contains hemorrhage in various stages and is surrounded by hemosiderin laden macrophages in the surrounding brain parenchyma. Typically these lesions produce seizure foci or focal neurologic deficit and, less commonly, headache. The lesions appear as iso- or hyper-dense inhomogeneous foci that have minimal to no associated contrast enhancement. There is frequently associated calcification within the lesion. There is usually no associated mass effect or edema. The lesions have a relatively characteristic appearance on MR imaging where they demonstrate inhomogeneous signal intensity with a surrounding hypointense rim resulting from hemosiderin deposition.

Venous Angiomas and Capillary Telangiectasias

The two remaining vascular malformations include venous angiomas and capillary telangiectasias. Neither of these lesions is a frequent cause of intracerebral hemorrhage. In fact, capillary telangiectasias usually have no associated symptoms, are all but invisible on CT imaging, and only sometimes can be visualized on contrast enhanced MR images. Venous angiomas, however, have a relatively characteristic appearance on contrast enhanced CT images, showing multiple tufts of enhancing vessels often near a ventricle being drained by a single collecting vein, producing a "Medusa head" appearance. Venous angiomas are a developmental abnormality and usually have no clinical significance.

Hemorrhage
Patient 5-1 • Intracerebral Hemorrhage

FIGURE 5-1 (Noncontrast)

The extremely large hyperdensity occupying the right basal ganglia is consistent with an acute intracerebral hemorrhage. There is associated contralateral midline shift and subfalcial herniation with severe hydrocephalus most evident in the area of the left temporal horn, which is markedly dilated. Hydrocephalus likely results from compression of the cerebral aqueduct. There is acute hemorrhage also demonstrated in the interhemispheric fissure anteriorly and is accompanied by acute intraventricular hemorrhage at the level of the third and fourth ventricles. The location of the hemorrhage within the basal ganglia is suggestive of a hypertensive origin but an aneurysm or vascular malformation can not be entirely excluded.

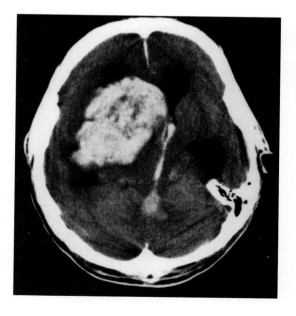

Patient 5-2 • Acute Intracerebral Hemorrhage

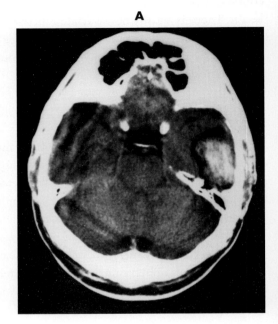

A

FIGURE 5-2, A (Noncontrast)

Homogeneous hyperdensity in the left temporal lobe consistent with acute intracerebral hemorrhage. This is indistinguishable from traumatic contusion based on CT findings alone.

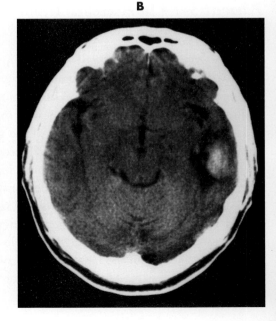

B

FIGURE 5-2, B (Noncontrast)

This image 10 mm higher shows the superior extent of the intracerebral hemorrhage. Its location posterior to the Sylvian fissure makes this less likely to represent an acute intracranial hemorrhage secondary to aneurysm rupture. The lack of acute subarachnoid hemorrhage also is atypical for aneurysm rupture. There is edema surrounding the blood clot and this finding generally is not seen with an extra axial (epidural and subdural) hematoma (see Figure 2-6, *A* and *B*).

Patient 5-3 • Cerebellar (Posterior Fossa) Hemorrhage

Noteworthy Point: It is important to recognize posterior fossa hemorrhage, since it is a true neurosurgical emergency with a good prognosis following emergent surgery.

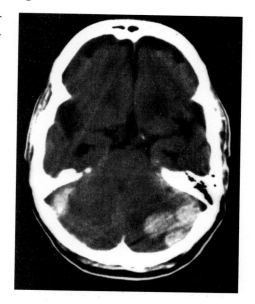

FIGURE 5-3 (Noncontrast)

This demonstrates a tri-lobed acute hemorrhage in the left cerebellar hemisphere with associated acute hemorrhage in the subarachnoid space of both cerebellopontine angle cisterns. Note the slight compression and distortion of the fourth ventricle, which is pushed slightly to the right.

Patient 5-4 • Intraparenchymal and Intraventricular Hemorrhage

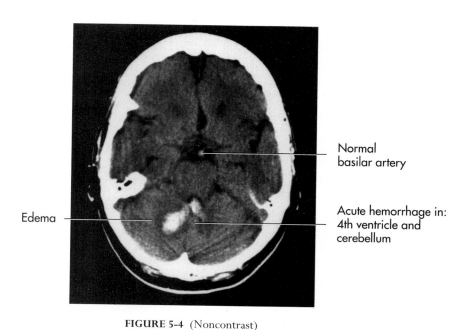

Normal
basilar artery

Edema

Acute hemorrhage in:
4th ventricle and
cerebellum

FIGURE 5-4 (Noncontrast)

Patient 5-5 • Cerebellar (Posterior Fossa) Hemorrhage

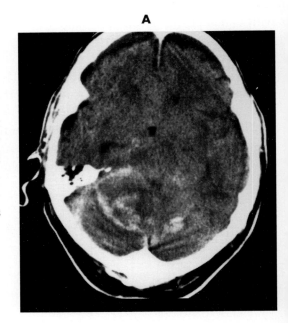

FIGURE 5-5, A (Noncontrast)

An ill-defined hyperdensity in the right cerebellar hemisphere is most consistent with an acute posterior fossa hemorrhage. There is also acute subarachnoid hemorrhage in the right cerebellopontine angle cistern evidenced by the peripheral curvilinear hyperdensity located lateral to the hemisphere. There is frontal atrophy.

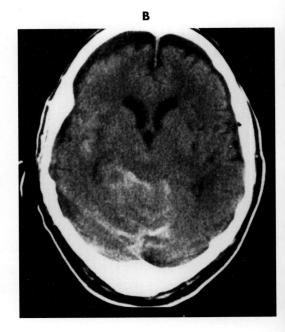

FIGURE 5-5, B (Noncontrast)

The acute subarachnoid hemorrhage is demonstrated within the sulci between the cerebellar folia and in the quadrigeminal plate cistern.

Patient 5-6 • Medulla Oblongata Hemorrhage

This case should serve as a reminder of the importance of examining the lower cuts on all CT scans.

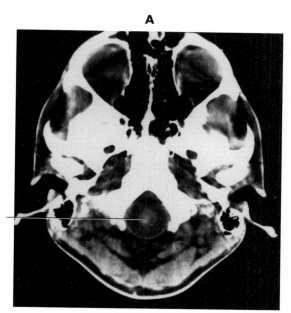

A

FIGURE 5-6, A (Noncontrast)

There is a small subtle hyperdensity in the medulla dorsally that may indicate the presence of a small intramedullary acute hemorrhage.

Hemorrhage

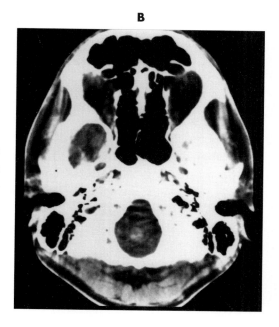

B

FIGURE 5-6, B (Noncontrast)

This demonstrates the superior extent of the medullary hemorrhage as a subtle hyperdensity. This was confirmed to represent acute hemorrhage by a subsequently performed MRI examination of the brain.

Arteriovenous Malformation (AVM)

Patient 5-7 • AVM

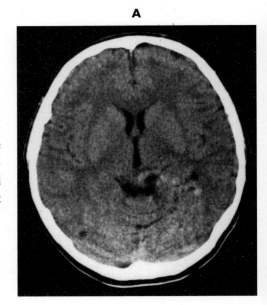

A

FIGURE 5-7, A (Noncontrast)

This demonstrates subtle hyperdensities in the left posterior temporal region, some with a serpiginous nature but without significant mass effect. The appearance is suggestive of an arteriovenous malformation with enlarged feeding arteries and draining veins. Figure 5-7, *C*, is a cut at the same level after contrast infusion.

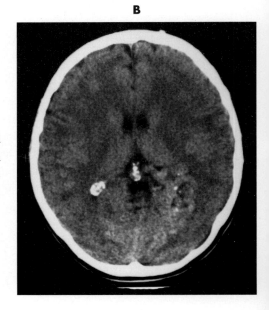

B

FIGURE 5-7, B (Noncontrast)

The serpiginous hyperdensities, some with associated calcification, in the left posterior temporal region are again most consistent with an arteriovenous malformation. Figure 5-7, *D*, is a cut at the same level after contrast infusion.

C

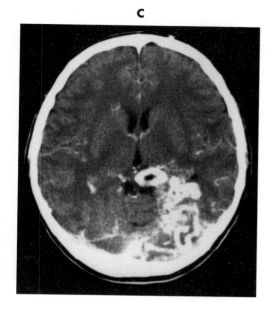

FIGURE 5-7, C (Contrast enhanced)

This shows multiple contrast enhancing serpiginous hyperdensities consistent with enhancing vessels and a large arteriovenous malformation that involves the left posterior temporal and the occipital region. The largest hyperdensity located near the anterior margin is an enlarged draining vein leading to the deep venous system.

D

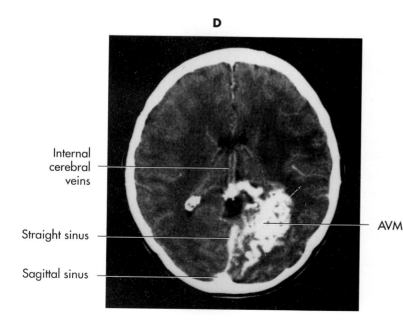

Internal
cerebral
veins

Straight sinus

Sagittal sinus

AVM

FIGURE 5-7, D (Contrast Enhanced)

This cut 10 mm higher shows the superior extent of the arteriovenous malformation and the enlarged draining vein leading to the deep venous system near its anterior and medial margin.

Patient 5-8 • AVM

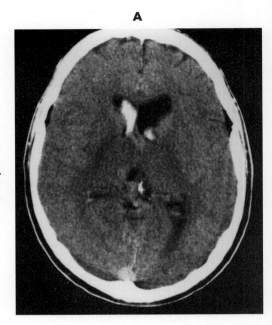

A

FIGURE 5-8, A (Noncontrast)

There is acute intraventricular hemorrhage in the area of the frontal horns particularly on the right. An ill-defined subtle hyperdensity is suspected in the area of the third ventricle extending posteriorly to the level of the pineal gland.

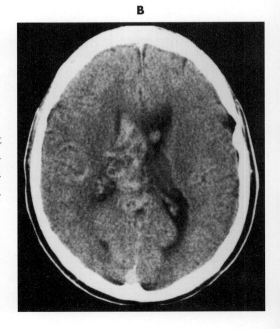

B

FIGURE 5-8, B (Noncontrast)

This cut 10 mm superiorly demonstrates a somewhat inhomogeneous ill-defined space occupying lesion, portions of which appear serpiginous in nature. The appearance is suggestive of a large midline arteriovenous malformation.

Patient 5-9 • Cavernous Angioma

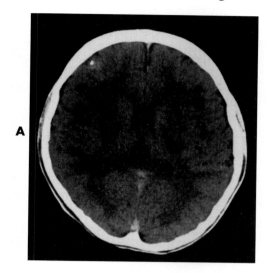

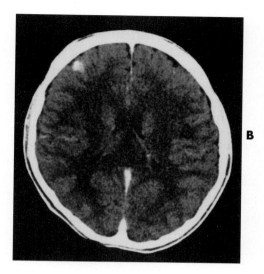

FIGURE 5-9, A (Noncontrast)

A punctate hyperdensity consistent with a focal calcification in the right frontal lobe is surrounded by an area of subtle hyperdensity that blends into the normal gray matter.

FIGURE 5-9, B (Contrast enhanced)

This demonstrates that the area surrounding the focal calcification shows some contrast enhancement but no mass effect or surrounding edema in this slice. The appearance is most consistent with a solitary cavernous angioma. This was confirmed on MRI imaging. See p. 104.

Patient 5-10 • Cavernous Angioma

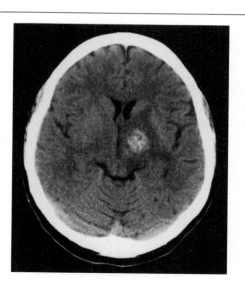

FIGURE 5-10 (Noncontrast)

A relatively large slightly inhomogeneous hyperdensity is present in the left thalamus. The density is typical for a cavernous angioma. The large size and surrounding edema (related to recent internal hemorrhage) are atypical.

Patient 5-11 • Venous Angioma

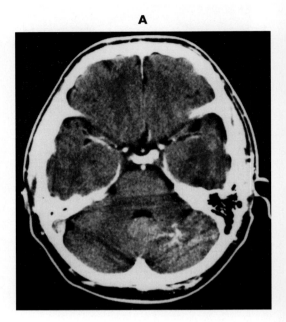

A

FIGURE 5-11, A (Contrast Enhanced)

An intraparenchymal hyperdensity consistent with abnormal enhancement is present in the area of the left middle cerebellar peduncle and left cerebellar hemisphere.

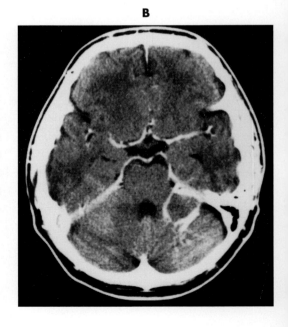

B

FIGURE 5-11, B (Contrast Enhanced)

This image obtained 5 mm more superiorly demonstrates that the ill-defined areas of enhancement are associated with two linear hyperdensities extending to the area of the left sigmoid sinus. The appearance is consistent with multiple collector veins with two large laterally draining veins that in combination are consistent with a diagnosis of venous angioma. See p. 105.

CHAPTER 6

INTRACRANIAL NEOPLASMS

This topic has an enormous scope, which must be limited for the purposes of this book. Large neoplastic lesions requiring emergency intervention are usually quite apparent on CT scan and are readily appreciated. However, although clinicians may have some anxiety about overlooking subtle CT findings of neoplasms, these rarely require emergency intervention and will be diagnosed by the radiologist during the official interpretation. In contrast, traumatic lesions, acute SAH, and strokes must be identified on CT images in the emergency department, and the subtle CT findings of these conditions are illustrated in earlier chapters. This chapter provides examples of the more common tumors and, hopefully, a way to help organize the information gleaned from the CT images of a patient with a space occupying lesion.

In the emergency department, the interpretation of a cranial CT scan that demonstrates a space occupying lesion is not that of providing an accurate histologic diagnosis, which is not always possible even after biopsy, but rather to accurately describe, locate, and give a short differential diagnosis of possibilities if the imaging features are in keeping with a neoplastic process.

Tumors can conveniently be grouped into those involving the brain (intra-axial in location) and those arising from the coverings of the brain, i.e., the meninges or ventricles (extra-axial in location).

In the first section of this chapter, a few brief comments about some of the tumors are presented. Table 6-1 provides an overview of the tumor images that are reproduced here and summarizes their CT features. However, neither a classification system nor a comprehensive discussion are intended.

Extra-Axial Tumors
Meningiomas

Extra-axial tumors arising from the meninges are most commonly meningiomas. These tumors usually are isodense to gray matter, intensely enhance, and usually have a broad base of attachment to the meninges. Meningiomas can arise from any portion of the meninges but are most common in areas of dural reflection (see Table 6-1). Accompanying edema of the underlying brain parenchyma can often be present. Metastatic disease to the meninges is usually in the form of meningeal carcinomatosis. Nodular meningeal deposits can also be seen but these are usually considerably smaller than meningiomas.

Ventricles

In adults intraventricular tumors are relatively rare and are more common in the supratentorial compartment, compared to children in whom a fourth ventricular location is most common. Differential diagnosis of supratentorial intraventricular tumors includes meningiomas, colloid cyst, choroid plexus papillomas, carcinomas, ependymomas, and metastases. Intraventricular tumors in the area of the fourth ventricle and cerebellar vermis are more common in children and a differential diagnosis includes medulloblastoma, ependymoma, and cerebellar cystic astrocytoma. These are best differentiated on CT images based on their precontrast densities, with medulloblastomas being the most dense, cerebellar astrocytomas least dense, and ependymomas intermediate between the two.

Intra-Axial Tumors
Gliomas (also called astrocytomas)

Of all intra-axial tumors the most common primary tumors are gliomas. These characteristically present with seizures. These lesions typically demonstrate a hypodense appearance relative to surrounding gray matter in which they arise and may or may not have surrounding edema extending into the subjacent white matter. If there is associated contrast enhancement, this indicates that the glioma is of a higher grade, at least grade III to IV. Lower grade gliomas generally do not enhance.

Aggressive high grade gliomas unassociated with pre-existing lower grade gliomas are usually termed *glioblastoma multiforme*. Gliomas with associated calcific components arising mainly in the frontal or temporal regions are more likely to represent oligodendrogliomas. Gliomas arising in the mesial temporal region in children or young adults with cystic or calcific components may represent a ganglioglioma. Ependymomas previously mentioned as intraventricular masses can occur intra-axially and are indistinguishable from gliomas, to which they are related. Gliomas tend to have a tendency to infiltrate adjacent brain parenchyma and if this is extensive, with what appears to be a low grade glioma, a diagnosis of gliomatosis cerebri should be considered. If there is evidence of an aggressive high grade glioma and there is infiltration of the corpus callosum, this may extend to the contralateral cerebral hemisphere, producing a typical "butterfly" appearance.

Lymphomas

Lymphomas frequently involve the brain and typically involve the subependymal region, where isodense nodules show intense contrast enhancement and are surrounded by edema. Lymphomas may also present as irregular inhomogeneous enhancing masses, indistinguishable from high grade gliomas both by their appearance and their tendency to involve the corpus callosum.

Tumors of specific areas

A differential diagnosis of tumors involving specific areas of the cranium is more limited and more specific. Three areas will be discussed: the suprasellar region, the cerebellopontine angle cistern region, and the third ventricle.

Suprasellar

In the suprasellar region the most likely mass identified is that of a pituitary macroadenoma with suprasellar extension. *Careful review of the scout film usually identifies an enlarged sella turcica.* One should also consider the possibility of a craniopharyngioma: these are usually inhomogeneous with calcific solid and cystic components and usually have a normal sella on the scout view. Other possibilities include suprasellar metastasis, suprasellar meningiomas (which can also arise from the adjacent cavernous sinus), gliomas of the optic chiasm or hypothalamus, and suprasellar aneurysms, which, in the case of a suprasellar enhancing mass on CT, must always be excluded with an MRI examination and/or angiographic study.

Cerebellopontine angle tumors

In the cerebellopontine angle (CPA) cistern there are three major differential diagnoses to consider. The first two are hyperdense and include meningioma and acoustic neurinoma. The third is the epidermoid, which is usually hypodense with a lobulated appearance and often extends into the middle cranial fossa. Arachnoid cysts can arise in this region also and have a hypodense appearance but are sharper in their outline and contain no internal septations.

Third ventricle

When there is a mass in the area of the third ventricle one must differentiate between an anterior intraventricular mass causing obstruction at the foramen of Munro and a ventricular lesion in the area of the aqueduct of Sylvius with associated dilatation of the third ventricle.

An isolated anterior intraventricular mass with associated obstructive hydrocephalus confined to the lateral ventricles would most likely represent a benign tumor known as a *colloid cyst*. These may be hyperdense or hypodense. Colloid cysts typically are associated with headache that often depends on specific head positions due to intermittent worsening of hydrocephalus as a result of movement of the colloid cyst within the ventricle itself.

Hydrocephalus involving the lateral ventricles and the third ventricle implies a mass near the posterior portion of the third ventricle or more likely near its outlet at the level of the aqueduct of Sylvius. This could be the result of congenital aqueductal stenosis, the most common cause of isolated hydrocephalus in children (Figure 8-2, *A*). Alternatively, it could be the result of compression of the aqueduct of Sylvius by masses arising from the overlying structures of the quadrigeminal plate or pineal gland. These include tectal gliomas and pineal tumors respectively. The pineal tumors include the germ cell variety most commonly seen in males and pineal cell-type tumors most commonly seen in females. Other masses involving the pineal gland include metastasis.

Metastases

Cerebral metastases account for approximately one third of all intracerebral neoplasms. These often are the first presenting sign of an underlying but yet unknown primary malignancy. Metastases may be intra or extra axial. A very large percentage of solitary intracranial tumors are metastases rather than primary tumors.

The most common cerebral metastases are small cell and adenocarcinoma of the lung and breast carcinoma. Renal cell, colon carcinoma, and melanoma are the next most common group of cerebral metastases.

Metastases typically are nodular or ring enhancing in character, often with surrounding edema, particularly when the lesions reach a certain size, and are frequent in the posterior fossa as well as the supratentorial compartment. Associated calcifications may indicate a mucinous carcinoma as the primary tumor. Extremely thin-walled ring enhancing lesions are suggestive of squamous cell carcinoma as the primary tumor—often from the head and neck in men and genitourinary tract in women.

CT Characteristics of Tumors

Table 6-1 summarizes the CT characteristics of tumors and provides references to the atlas images for the examples that are included in the image section, which follows. The captions and labels accompanying the images elaborate on the above introduction.

NOTE: The images are arranged in the order indicated in Table 6-1.

TABLE 6-1   CT characteristics of tumors

Tumor	Density Relative to Gray Matter on Unenhanced CT	Enhances	Favored Location	Other Features
Extra-Axial				
Meningioma Figure 6-1 and 6-2	Hyper or isodense	Intensely	Areas of dural reflection, particularly: Convex areas Suprasellar Cavernous sinus CP angle Intraventricular	
Acoustic neurinoma Figure 6-4	Isodense	Moderate to intense	Cerebellopontine angle cistern Internal auditory canal	Widened internal auditory canal Inhomogeneous density
Pituitary adenoma Figure 6-5	Iso to hypodense to pituitary	Less than normal gland tissue	Sella Suprasellar	Enlarged pituitary fossa (examine on scout view) Erosion of floor of pituitary fossa
Metastases Figures 6-6 and 6-7	Isodense	Usually intense	Dural based	Often has associated intra-axial edema
Extra-Axial and Intraventricular				
Medulloblastoma	Hyperdense	Little	Fourth ventricle	Arises from cerebellar vermis
Colloid cyst Figures 6-8 to 6-10	Hyperdense Occassionally hypodense	Little	Anterior third ventricle	Often with obstructive hydrocephalus of lateral ventricles
Ependymoma Figure 6-11	Isodense	Mild to moderate	Fourth ventricle	May have intra- and extra-axial location Fifty percent are calcified Often extends to cerebellopontine angle cistern and thru foramen magnum
Cerebellar astrocytoma Figure 6-12	Hypodense	None	Fourth ventricle	Often cystic in appearance
Metastases	Isodense	Usually intense		
Intra-Axial				
Glioma Figures 6-13 to 6-17	Hypodense	None/low/ inhomogeneous High	Hemispheres Brainstem	If calcified and frontal or temporal, consider oligodendroglioma
Lymphoma Figure 6-19	Iso to hypodense	Intense	Periventricular	In HIV patients may have atypical appearance resembling glioma
Hemangioblastomas Figure 6-20	Cystic, hypo or isodense; have a nodule	Nodule enhances intensely	Posterior fossa	Classically has a big cyst and a small nodule Multiple in Von Hippel-Lindau
Metastases Figures 6-21 to 6-25	Iso to hypodense	Usually intense	Cortical-subcortical junction	May be ring enhancing, especially squamous cell carcinomas

Extra-Axial Tumors

MENINGIOMAS

Patient 6-1 • Meningioma

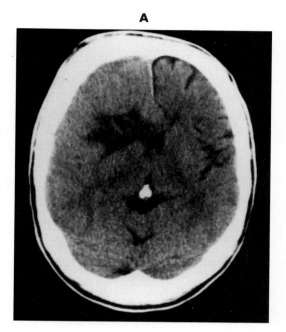

FIGURE 6-1, *A* (Noncontrast)

The most obvious abnormality is the hypodense change in the subcortical region of the right frontal lobe with associated mass effect distorting the frontal horns and producing slight shift to the left. This, however, is not the main abnormality. The main abnormality is a right frontal mass obliterating the gray-white junction and the cortical sulci. This slightly hyperdense mass abuts the falx and is most likely a meningioma.

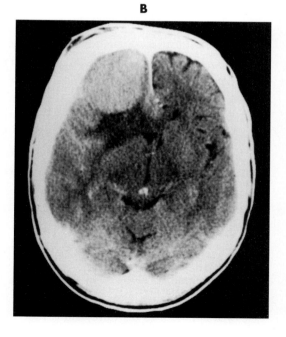

FIGURE 6-1, *B* (Contrast enhanced)

After contrast enhancement the mass is clearly identified as hyperdense, indicating marked enhancement. This is contiguous with the dural reflection over the right convexity and the right side of the falx. These findings confirm that this is a convexity meningioma with subjacent subcortical edema.

Patient 6-2 • Meningioma

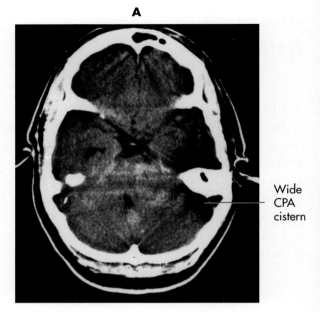

A

FIGURE 6-2, *A* (Noncontrast)

A subtle isodense to slightly hyperdense mass is present in the left cerebellopontine angle (CPA) cistern, causing this cistern to appear abnormally wide. The mass distorts the left lateral aspect of the fourth ventricle and pushes this ventricle to the right.

Wide
CPA
cistern

FIGURE 6-2, *B* (Contrast enhanced)

This enhanced scan is at the same level as Figure 6-2, *A*. The space occupying lesion enhances intensely and is seen to have a wide dural base of attachment along the tentorium. On Figure 6-2, *A*, this mass can be faintly seen, even without contrast enhancement—the wide CPA cistern is the clue to the existence of this mass even though the hypodensity of the cistern tricks the eye, making the mass difficult to perceive.

The bone windows (not shown) demonstrate that the internal auditory canal (IAC) is normal (distortion of this structure is expected in the case of an acoustic neurinoma).

This appearance is classic for meningioma because: (1) of the location of the lesion, (2) the fact that it has a broad base of attachment to the dura, and (3) the IAC is normal.

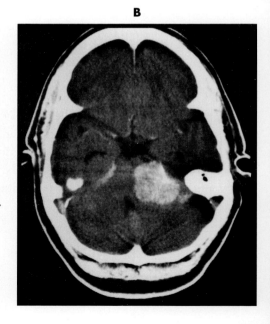

B

Patient 6-3 • CPA Tumor (L)

A

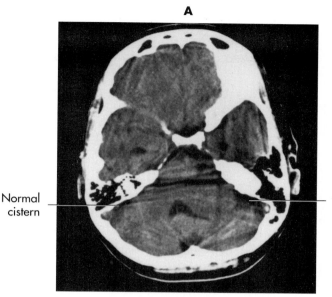

FIGURE 6-3, *A* (Noncontrast)

The main clue to the presence of a tumor is the mass effect on the lateral aspect of the fourth ventricle, which causes it to be bowed in a concave manner. This is most likely to be extra-axial in location due to the associated widening of the left cerebellopontine angle cistern. It is not possible to determine exactly which type of tumor this is, based on this CT alone.

Normal cistern

Wide CPA cistern

B

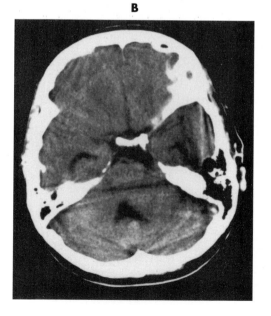

FIGURE 6-3, *B* (Noncontrast)

This cut immediately above the previous cut again demonstrates widening of the left cerebellopontine angle cistern and distortion of the left lateral aspect of the fourth ventricle. Compression of the outlet of the fourth ventricle caused obstructive hydrocephalus, as evidenced by the enlarged temporal horns and the prominent fourth ventricle.

Patient 6-4 • Acoustic Neurinoma

FIGURE 6-4, *A* (Contrast enhanced)

A

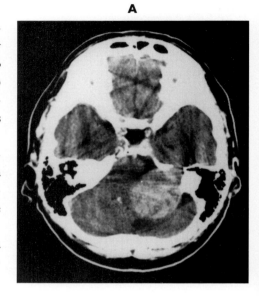

The left internal auditory canal (IAC) is enlarged and distorted—this is not a finding related to possible asymmetry of the cut. A large homogeneously enhancing mass is seen to exit from the IAC and fills the cerebellopontine angle (CPA) cistern. The cerebellum and fourth ventricle are compressed. The CPA cistern is enlarged, which defines this as an extra-axial tumor.

The features that define this mass as an acoustic neurinoma rather than a meningioma are: (1) this mass has a shorter dural base than is seen with a meningioma (see Figure 6-2, *B*), (2) the apex is located in the IAC, and (3) the IAC is distorted.

Most acoustic neurinomas are now diagnosed earlier on a contrast enhanced MRI, often when the tumor is still confined within the IAC.

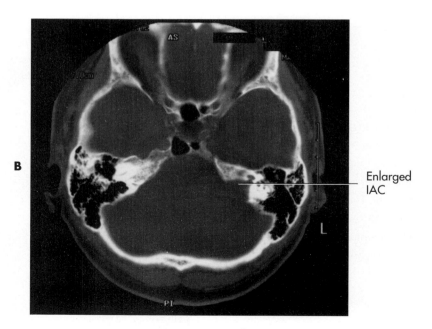

Enlarged
IAC

FIGURE 6-4, *B* (Bone window)

PITUITARY ADENOMA

Patient 6-5 • Empty Sella

FIGURE 6-5 (Scout view)

This case stresses the importance of examining the scout view. There is marked enlargement of the pituitary fossa with thinning of the dorsum sella but no obvious focal bony erosion. Compare to the normal sized pituitary fossa in Figure 1-8, A, and Figure 2-27, C. Causes of an enlarged sella include: pituitary adenoma, primary empty sella, and long standing hydrocephalus.

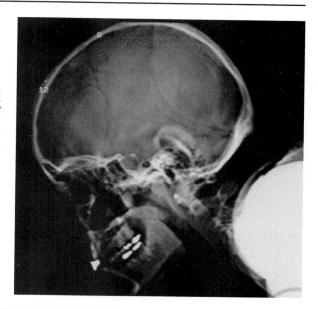

METASTASES (EXTRA-AXIAL)

Patient 6-6 • Metastases to Skull or Subjacent Meninges

Isodense mass with cortical effacement

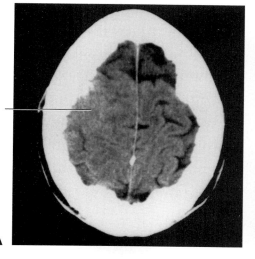

A

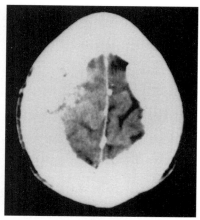

B

FIGURE 6-6, *A* **and** *B* (Noncontrast)

The subtle cortical effacement in the right frontal cortex is due to mass effect and is an important clue to the adjacent inhomogeneous isodense space occupying lesion. This is associated with spiculated calcification or ossification that blends with the adjacent inner table of the skull.

Continued

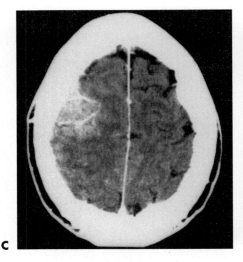
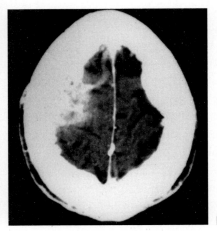

C

D

FIGURE 6-6 cont'd, *C* **and** *D* (Contrast enhanced)

The lesion contrast enhances and appears to arise from the meninges or overlying skull vault. Most likely this represents a metastatic malignant neoplasm of the skull or subjacent meninges but the differential includes a primary bone malignancy such as osteosarcoma. The final pathology was metastasis from the known bowel carcinoma. There is a prominent vein draining anteriorly from this region.

E

FIGURE 6-6, *E* (Bone window)

The skull is clearly eroded. Only an extra-axial mass could be responsible for this finding.

Bone erosion

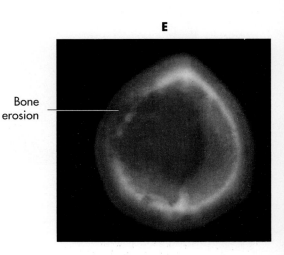

Patient 6-7 • Leptomeningeal Metastases

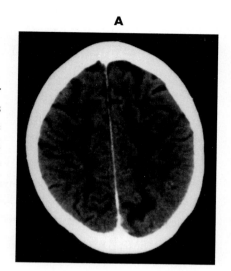

A

FIGURE 6-7, *A* (Contrast enhanced)

A serpiginous low density area is identified in the left posterior parietal subcortical white matter. There is also subtle local mass effect: note the loss of cortical sulci at the outer perimeter of the low density area. The pattern is atypical for acute ischemia and therefore raises the possibility of subcortical edema. Because no obvious brain abnormality on CT accounts for this edema an MRI was performed to search for abnormality at the level of the leptomeninges or skull.

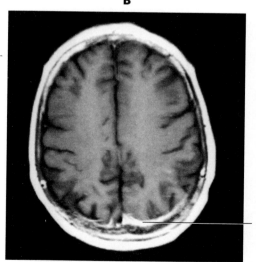

B

FIGURE 6-7, *B* (MRI head—contrast enhanced)

This T1W image demonstrates abnormal gadolinium enhancement involving the leptomeninges in the posterior parietal region with left sided predominance. This is compatible with meningeal based tumor, likely leptomeningeal metastases. The hypodense abnormality seen on the CT scan is reactive vasogenic edema.

Tumor

Extra-Axial And Intraventricular Tumors

COLLOID CYST

Patient 6-8 • Classic Colloid Cyst

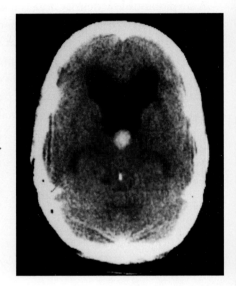

FIGURE 6-8 (Noncontrast)

This demonstrates a homogeneously hyperdense mass in the anterior third ventricle with marked dilatation of the lateral ventricles, particularly the frontal horns, due to obstruction of the third ventricle. The appearance is practically pathognomonic of a colloid cyst. These typically have a hyperdense appearance due to homogeneous, thick, highly proteinaceous material that fills them, although they can be hypodense (see Figure 6-9, *A*).

Patient 6-9 • Colloid Cyst

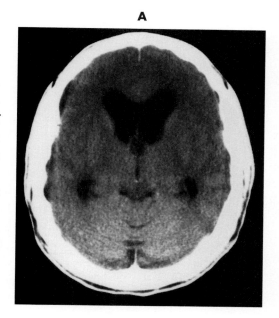

FIGURE 6-9, *A* (Noncontrast)

This image reveals the presence of a round hypo-dense space occupying lesion in the anterior third ventricle associated with an obstructive hydrocephalus of the lateral ventricles. The lesion may not be apparent without careful study of the image because it is in the midline but the hydrocephalus mandates such scrutiny. It is in the same position as the hyperdense colloid cyst seen on the noncontrast study, Figure 6-8. The appearance is most consistent with a colloid cyst. Colloid cysts may be hyper or hypo dense but are invariably located in the anterior third ventricle.

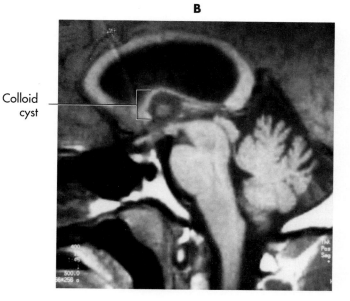

B

FIGURE 6-9, *B* (T1W sagittal MRI—noncontrast)

This MRI demonstrates the anterior third ventricular mass that displaces the fornices superiorly and has two components: a hypointense periphery and an iso-intense center. The higher signal intensity in the central component probably represents thick proteinaceous material.

Colloid cyst

Patient 6-10 • Colloid Cyst

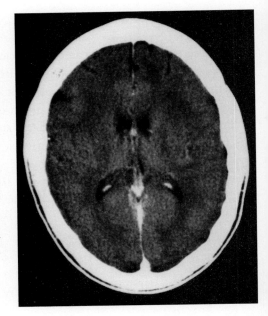

FIGURE 6-10 (Contrast enhanced)

This contrast enhanced CT image demonstrates a very small anterior third ventricular mass in the same location as the previous examples of colloid cyst. The hyperdensity could be the result of: (1) highly proteinaceous thick material or (2) the presence of abnormal contrast enhancement. A noncontrast study was not obtained but if the location and appearance were the same on a noncontrast study, this would be almost pathognomonic of a small colloid cyst. The small size was unassociated with the presence of hydrocephalus, which usually occurs later when there is obstruction of the foramen of Munro. MRI confirmed the diagnosis of colloid cyst.

EPENDYMOMA

Patient 6-11 • Ependymoma

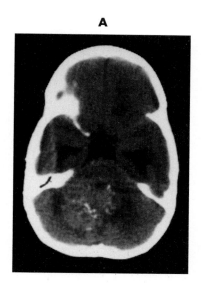

A

FIGURE 6-11, *A* (Noncontrast)

This demonstrates an isodense space occupying lesion in the area of the fourth ventricle with associated calcifications and a slight surrounding hypodense halo that probably represents edema. There is marked hydrocephalus. The isodensity of the mass and the associated calcification favors the diagnosis of ependymoma over astrocytoma or medulloblastoma.

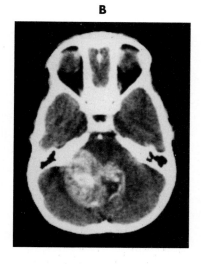

B

FIGURE 6-11, *B* (Contrast enhanced)

The marked but inhomogeneous contrast enhancement of the midline mass is seen to extend into the right cerebellopontine angle cistern. Extension through the basal foramina of the fourth ventricle or to the cerebellopontine angle cistern favors the diagnosis of ependymoma over medulloblastoma or astrocytoma.

Cerebellar Astrocytoma

Patient 6-12 • Cerebellar Astrocytoma

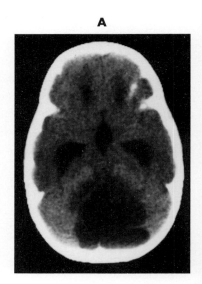

A

FIGURE 6-12, *A* (Noncontrast)

There is a very large lobulated mass in the area of the cerebellar vermis compressing the fourth ventricle and producing marked hydrocephalus. The mass is hypodense and apparently has a cystic component involving its posterior two thirds. The contrast enhanced study (not included) demonstrated very minimal enhancement.

This appearance is most consistent with the diagnosis of a cystic astrocytoma arising from the cerebellar vermis (fourth ventricular roof). The differential diagnosis would include medulloblastoma and ependymoma. However, medulloblastomas tend to be hyperdense before contrast enhancement and ependymomas are usually isodense.

B

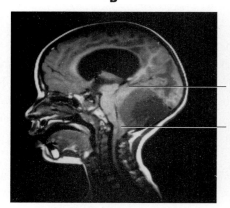

Cerebellar vermis

Cerebellar tonsil

FIGURE 6-12, *B* (MRI T1W sagittal)

The large posterior fossa mass is seen to have solid and cystic components. It arises from the cerebellar vermis and compresses the fourth ventricle. Note the superior herniation of the cerebellar vermis and inferior herniation of the cerebellar tonsils.

Intra-Axial Tumors

GLIOMAS (ASTROCYTOMAS)

Patient 6-13 • Low Grade Glioma

This demonstrates a hypodense space occupying lesion that does not enhance. It is located parasagittally on the right with a focal more profound hypodensity indicating an accompanying cystic component. This mass on other images (not shown) crosses vascular boundaries and is therefore more likely neoplastic rather than infarctive in nature. *The lack of contrast enhancement of the lesion indicates that it is relatively slow growing or nonmalignant.* Most likely this represents a low grade glioma with cystic components. A presenting history of seizures favors this diagnosis.

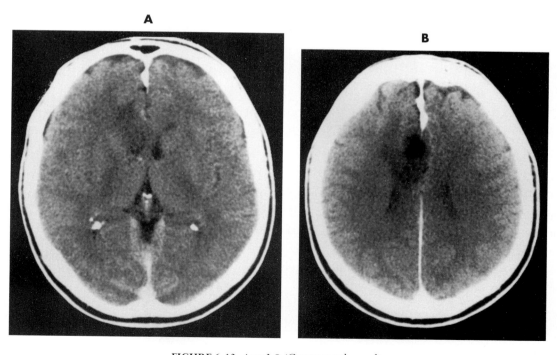

A   **B**

FIGURE 6-13, *A* **and** *B* (Contrast enhanced)

Patient 6-14 • Low Grade Glioma—Oligodendroglioma

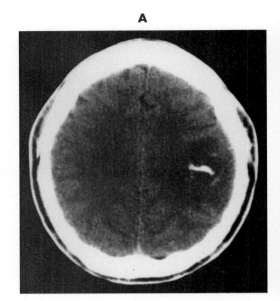

A

FIGURE 6-14, *A* (Noncontrast)

There is a left frontoparietal hypodense space occupying lesion with a linear central hyperdensity that has the appearance of calcification. Most likely this represents a neoplastic space occupying lesion; the associated calcification suggests a relatively benign or slow growing tumor. The presence of calcification makes oligodendroglioma the most likely diagnosis.

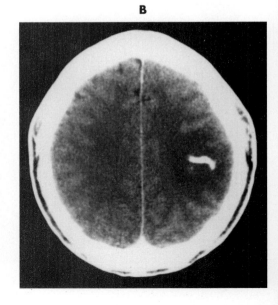

B

FIGURE 6-14, *B* (Contrast enhanced)

This demonstrates no associated enhancement in the lesion excluding an accompanying vascular malformation or a high grade component to the tumor. This therefore most likely represents a calcified low grade glioma and, of these, an oligodendroglioma is most likely. This was proven by biopsy.

Patient 6-15 • Glioblastoma Multiforme

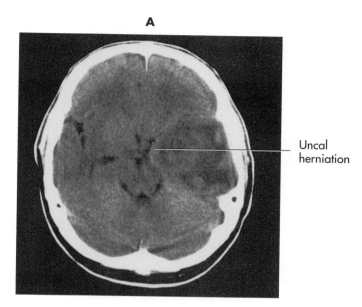

FIGURE 6-15, *A* (Noncontrast)

The inhomogeneous hypodense change in the left temporal region is suggestive of a space occupying lesion, probably neoplastic. There is low density surrounding edema and localized mass effect producing some left uncal herniation.

Uncal herniation

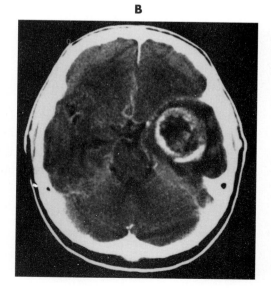

FIGURE 6-15, *B* (Contrast enhanced)

A contrast enhancing intra-axial space occupying lesion is evident. There is marked surrounding edema and anterior displacement of the left middle cerebral artery. The appearance is most consistent with a high grade glioma or glioblastoma multiforme (GBM) in view of the extensive inhomogeneous contrast enhancement and marked surrounding edema. The diagnosis of GBM was proven by biopsy.

Patient 6-16 • Glioblastoma Multiforme

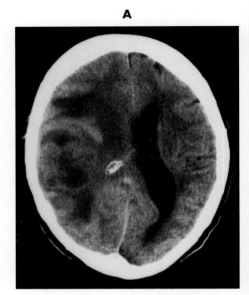

FIGURE 6-16, *A* (Noncontrast)

A large inhomogeneous space occupying lesion is present in the right frontal lobe. This has iso- and hypo-dense components and marked surrounding edema. The associated mass effect is producing: (1) marked compression of the ipsilateral lateral ventricle and (2) cortical sulci and contralateral midline shift with subfalcial herniation.

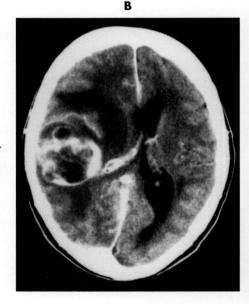

FIGURE 6-16, *B* (Contrast enhanced)

The mass demonstrates inhomogeneous contrast enhancement. Note the compressed and displaced choroid plexus of the right lateral ventricle. The appearance is consistent with a high grade glioma, most likely a glioblastoma multiforme.

Patient 6-17 • Glioblastoma Multiforme

FIGURE 6-17, *A* (noncontrast) and **B** (contrast enhanced)

An ill-defined primarily isodense space occupying lesion of both frontal lobes with surrounding edema is present. On the contrast enhanced image the lesion is seen to cross the corpus callosum and to enhance inhomogeneously. The appearance is highly suggestive for a very aggressive glioma such as a glioblastoma multiforme of the "butterfly" type.

The differential diagnosis would include only lymphoma. If one had the noncontrast study only, a diagnosis of cerebrovascular accident (CVA) should not be considered because: (1) the lesion is inhomogeneous in density, (2) the lesion is bilateral and would therefore have to involve the middle and anterior meningeal artery territories bilaterally, and (3) the lesion does not extend out to the cortex.

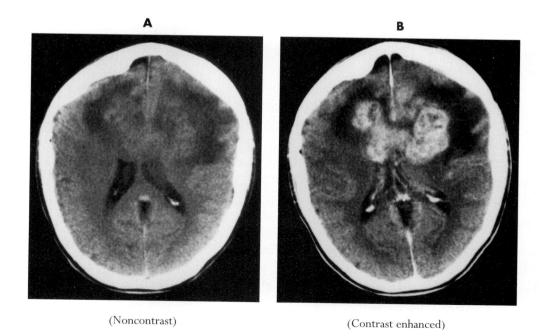

(Noncontrast)   (Contrast enhanced)

Patient 6-18 • High Grade Glioma versus Lymphoma

A

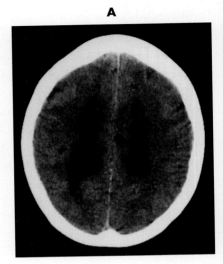

FIGURE 6-18, *A* (Noncontrast)

An inhomogeneous space occupying lesion is located above the roof of the third ventricle and between both lateral ventricles, indicating its location in the corpus callosum or in the overlying cingulate gyri. Not shown is surrounding edema on the slice immediately above.

B

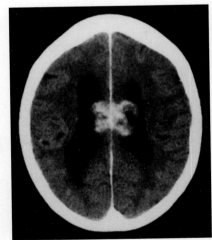

FIGURE 6-18, *B* (Contrast enhanced)

The previously demonstrated mass shows inhomogeneous but marked contrast enhancement, confirming its location and associated blood-brain barrier disruption. The differential diagnosis is basically between a high grade glioma crossing through the corpus callosum or a lymphoma.

Lymphoma

Patient 6-19 • Lymphoma

This is the typical appearance of a lymphoma in an immunocompetent patient. This patient, however, was HIV positive and, in general, immunocompromised patients may have atypical lymphomas that are indistinguishable from high grade gliomas on CT (see section on lymphomas above).

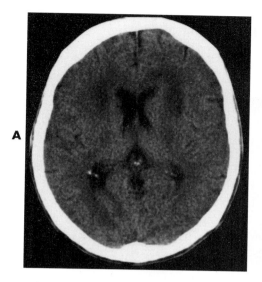

FIGURE 6-19, *A* (Noncontrast)

There is bilateral subcortical edema without an obvious cause for this finding on this image.

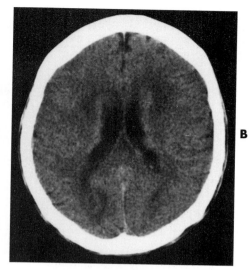

FIGURE 6-19, *B* (Noncontrast)

In addition to the bilateral edema, there is a suggestion of bilateral irregular masses involving the lateral walls of both ventricles.

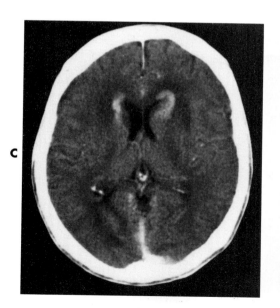

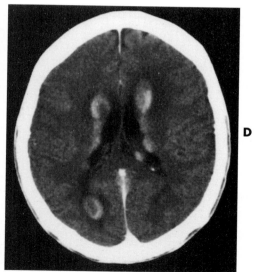

FIGURE 6-19, *C* and *D* (Contrast enhanced cuts at same level as A and B)

There is extensive enhancement of the walls of the lateral ventricles in the subependymal region. This appearance is highly suggestive of lymphoma.

Patient 6-20 • Hemangioblastoma

A

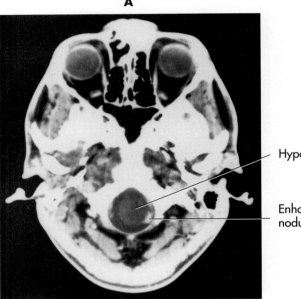

FIGURE 6-20, *A* (Contrast enhanced)

There is a subtle but definite hypodensity in the left lateral aspect of the medulla with a peripheral enhancing nodule in its wall. The typical CT appearance of hemangioblastomas is illustrated by this case: cystic masses of the posterior fossa with an enhancing mural nodule. However, this type of tumor involves the brainstem in less than 10% of cases because it is most commonly found in the cerebellum. This example emphasizes the importance of examining lower cuts of a CT study.

Hypodensity

Enhancing nodule

B

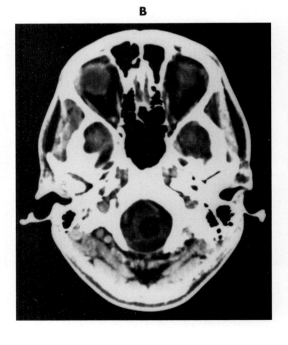

FIGURE 6-20, *B* (Contrast enhanced)

The hypodense, nonenhancing cystic portion of the tumor is seen again on the next higher cut. The enhancing nodule is not present at this level.

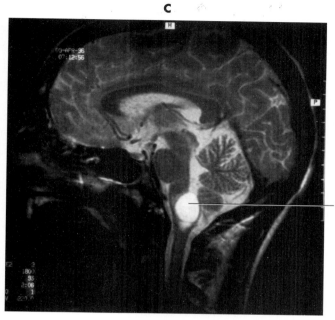

FIGURE 6-20, C
(T2W sagittal MRI—nonenhanced)

This demonstrates the cystic portion of the mass in the posterior aspect of the medulla just above the foramen magnum. The lesion appears very bright as the result of its highly proteinaceous composition.

Hemangio-
blastoma

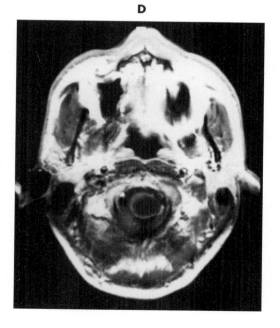

FIGURE 6-20, D (T1W axial MRI—contrast enhanced)

Demonstrated more clearly than on the CT are the cystic nature of the mass within the medulla on the left and the enhancing mural nodule on its extreme left lateral aspect.

METASTASES (Intra-axial)

Patient 6-21 • Metastatic Small Cell Carcinoma of Lung

There are innumerable contrast enhancing space occupying lesions at the cortical-subcortical junction supratentorially, in the basal ganglia, and in the cerebellum. There is no significant surrounding edema or significant mass effect. The lack of edema is often a feature of small and innumerable metastases. The cortical-subcortical location of the supratentorial lesions is fairly typical for metastasis because they lodge in the end arteries and arterioles.

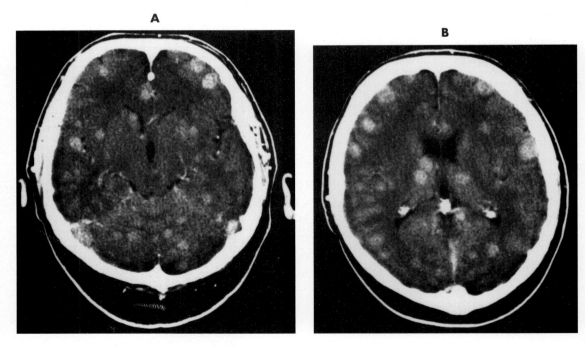

FIGURE 6-21, *A* and *B* (Contrast enhanced)

Patient 6-22 • Metastatic Bronchoalveolar Carcinoma

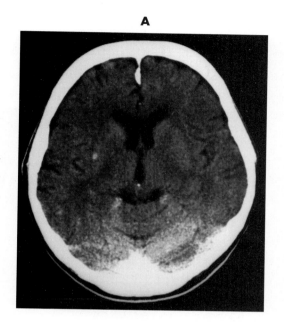

FIGURE 6-22, *A* (Contrast enhanced)

There are very subtle nodular hyperdensities identified in the right lentiform nucleus and in the right posterior temporal region at the cortical-subcortical junction.

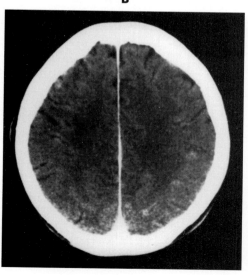

FIGURE 6-22, *B* (Contrast enhanced)

Multiple additional nodular hyperdensities are seen at the cortical-subcortical junction of both cerebral hemispheres, particularly in the parietal regions. In the absence of trauma, nodular hyperdensities on a contrast enhanced study suggest multiple areas of blood-brain barrier disruption. The lack of edema is unusual for cerebral abscesses; therefore in a patient with a previous history of carcinoma these are most likely early cerebral metastases.

The noncontrast study (not shown) appeared normal.

Continued

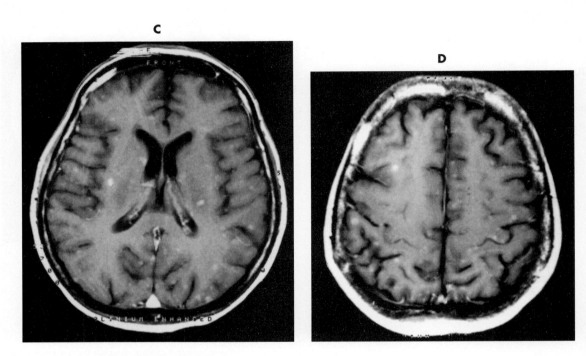

C

D

FIGURE 6-22, *C* and *D* (MRI—contrast enhanced)

These T1W images confirm the CT findings and reveal multiple nodular hyperdensities in keeping with focal contrast enhancement.

In the clinical setting this is compatible with multiple tiny cerebral metastasis.

Patient 6-23 • Hemorrhagic Metastases

FIGURE 6-23, *A* and *B* (Noncontrast)

This demonstrates at least three hyperdense, presumably hemorrhagic lesions with surrounding edema involving the left basal ganglia in Figure 6-23, *A*, and left frontal lobe parasagittally and in the opercular region on Figure 6-23, *B*. The surrounding edema and multiplicity of the lesions in the absence of trauma is suspicious for multiple neoplasms with internal hemorrhage and, as such, metastases would be the most likely cause. This patient had melanoma.

Noteworthy Point: Hemorrhagic neoplasms are seen most commonly in renal, thyroid, melanoma, and choriocarcinoma metastases.

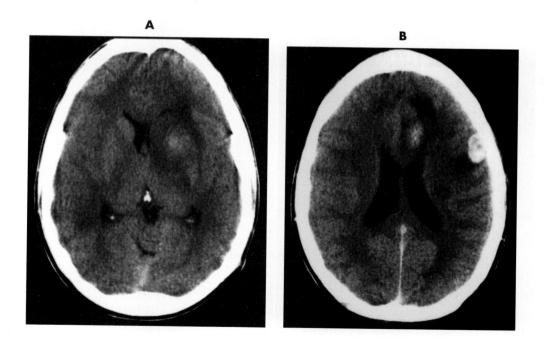

A

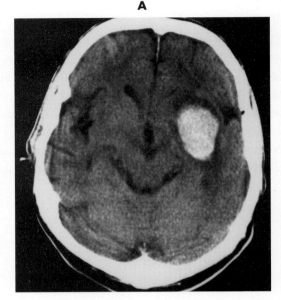

FIGURE 6-24, *A* (Noncontrast)

A homogenous hyperdensity in the left basal ganglia with surrounding edema. The differential diagnosis based solely on this image is acute intracerebral hemorrhage or possibly a hemorrhagic neoplasm.

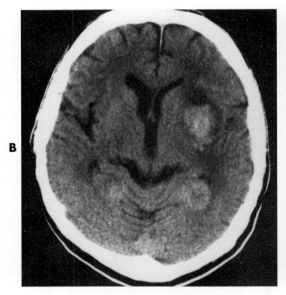

B

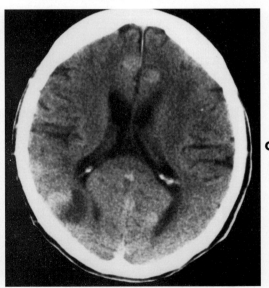

C

FIGURE 6-24, *B* and *C* (Noncontrast)

Additional intra-axial hyperdensities in the frontal lobes and right posterior parietal lobe. The posterior parietal lobe lesion has a region of surrounding hypodensity medially and this is most likely due to accompanying edema. These additional, albeit less, hyperdense intra-axial abnormalities, raise the possibility of cerebral metastases. The hyperdense components probably indicate accompanying internal hemorrhage that is most prominent in the left basal ganglia. The patient had known small cell carcinoma of the lung.

Patient 6-25 • Metastatic Small Cell Carcinoma of the Lung with Obstruction of the Aqueduct of Sylvius

FIGURE 6-25, *A-C* (Contrast enhanced)

There are multiple small contrast enhancing nodules. Most are at the cortical-subcortical junction. There is hydrocephalus, which is secondary to a metastatic lesion in the brainstem compressing the aqueduct.

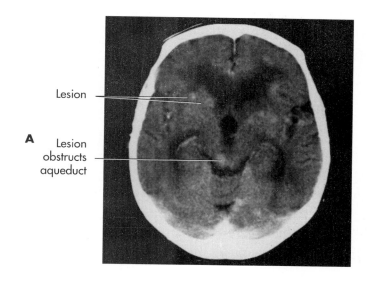

Lesion —

A Lesion
obstructs —
aqueduct

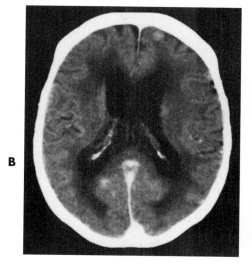

B

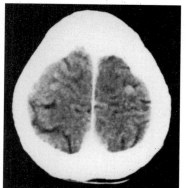

C

Continued

FIGURE 6-25, _D_ (MRI contrast enhanced)

This T1W axial MRI demonstrates the hydrocephalus and the enhancing metastatic nodule compressing the aqueduct.

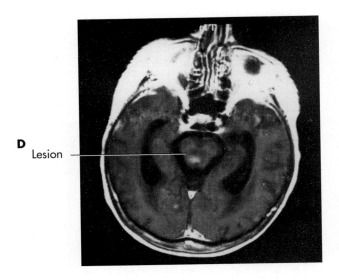

D
Lesion ——————

CHAPTER 7

Intracranial Infections

Chronic Infections

Chronic infections, particularly those that develop in utero or in the perinatal period, usually manifest as abnormal intracranial calcifications. These calcifications are usually in the periventricular regions and are more prominent than the physiologic calcifications usually seen in the globus pallidus region of the basal ganglia or the dentate nuclei of the cerebellum. Infections typically causing these periventricular calcifications belong to the TORCH series, particularly toxoplasmosis and cytomegalovirus.

Parasitic Infections

Certain types of infection, particularly of the parasitic variety, can be associated with calcifications and abnormal contrast enhancement. The best example of this is neurocysticercosis, whose larvae demonstrate a punctate calcification in the scolex when they become nonviable and often incite reaction in the surrounding brain in the form of a ring enhancing lesion with a central calcification.

Bacterial Infections

Most bacterial infections of the brain manifest as cerebritis. This is a rapidly developing and evolving ill-defined infection of the brain parenchyma following the deposition and crossing of a blood-brain barrier of bacterial organisms deposited in end arteries. The appearance is one of predominantly low density change, often in association with areas of patchy enhancement and accompanying edema and local mass effect. In the absence of appropriate therapy, cerebritis usually progresses to brain abscess formation in one to two weeks. The brain abscess is a more circumscribed abnormality that demonstrates a relatively thin enhancing wall that is smooth compared to the thicker, more irregular wall of a tumor. The abscess wall may be defective on its medial border due to a rapid growth and outstripping of the blood supply of the wall itself. This enhancing wall is composed of fibrin and may actually be useful in delineating the infective process from relatively normal but edematous surrounding brain if neurosurgical intervention is contemplated.

In addition to cerebritis and abscess formation, bacterial infections can be confined to the meninges and therefore produce a meningitis. The CT imaging manifestations of meningitis are nonspecific and usually include a communicating hydrocephalus and associated effaced cortical sulci. Abnormal enhancement of the meninges is not reliably detected on CT images because enhancement and the adjacent inner table of the skull are hyperdense. The radiologic features of meningitis are best demonstrated on gadolinium enhanced T1W MR images.

Bacterial infection confined to an end artery without blood-brain barrier disruption may be manifest in the development of an atypical "mycotic" aneurysm. These typically appear as peripheral enhancing nodules and may or may not have slight surrounding edema. A search for underlying bacterial endocarditis should be undertaken and cerebral angiography is required for definitive diagnosis.

Bacterial infections in the paranasal sinuses or mastoids may erode the inner table of the skull and spread to the adjacent subdural space. This results in a subdural empyema. This typically has the appearance of an isodense subdural fluid accumulation that shows peripheral enhancement in the involved subdural space. Because the infection is in the subdural space the infection can cross suture lines but never crosses the midline. It may spread inferiorly to involve the tentorium cerebelli if it arises primarily in the supratentorial compartment.

Atypical bacteria may involve the brain and its coverings and this is most commonly seen with infections of a tuberculous origin. Typically these patients manifest with a communicating hydrocephalus secondary to plugging of the arachnoid granulations, and there may be some prominent enhancement detected at the level of the meninges, particularly in the basal regions. Focal nodular abnormal enhancement may be seen usually adjacent to the basal cisterns in the form of accompanying tuberculomas.

Viral Infections

Viruses can affect the brain and its coverings, and when acute they are most likely the result of a herpes simplex infection. This agent causes herpes simplex encephalitis and manifests on CT scan as a hypodense, often patchy, area with accompanying edema seen most frequently in the temporal regions. This can be bilateral but more likely is unilateral and may be accompanied by patchy or mild contrast enhancement.

The combination of low density change and mild contrast enhancement may mask this condition and the diagnosis may be missed if a plain CT scan is not performed before contrast enhancement. However, in many cases of herpes encephalitis the CT scan will be normal and the purpose of the emergency CT is to rule out other neurologic emergencies. If the clinical suspicion of herpes encephalitis is strong, further investigation with MRI is necessary.

Viruses that involve the meninges can produce similar changes to a bacterial meningitis, although these are usually radiologically more mild and usually consist of a normal scan or very mild communicating hydrocephalus.

Intracranial Infections
Patient 7-1 • Cerebral Abscess

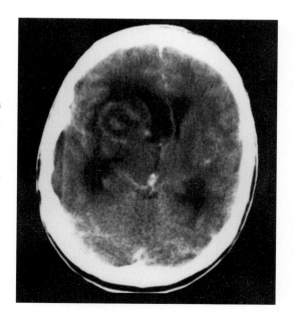

FIGURE 7-1 (Contrast enhanced)

This demonstrates a thin, ring-enhancing lesion with an area of central enhancement. There is marked surrounding edema and mass effect producing contralateral midline shift, subfalcial herniation, and hydrocephalus. The lack of enhancement of the ring in its medial border is quite suggestive of a cerebral abscess. This finding is thought to be the result of the abscess outstripping its blood supply due to rapid development.

Patient 7-2 • Cerebral Abscess

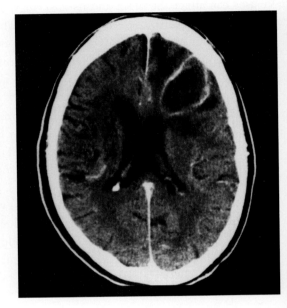

FIGURE 7-2 (Contrast enhanced)

A ring-enhancing space occupying lesion in the left frontal lobe is present. The ring enhancement is relatively thin and smooth in appearance and there is marked surrounding edema. Because of the thin wall, this appearance is more suggestive of an abscess than a neoplastic space occupying lesion (see the thick wall in Figure 6-15, *B*). A similar appearance could be expected in a resolving hematoma but some central hyperdensity may often persist in a resolving hematoma (see Figure 2-26, *A*).

Patient 7-3 • Subdural Empyema

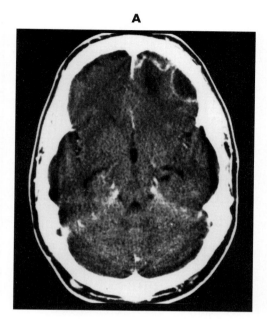

FIGURE 7-3, *A* (Contrast enhanced)

A semicircular type enhancing abnormality in the left frontal region abuts the meninges and inner table of the skull. The thin wall suggests an abscess. Because of its apparent dural base, this is most likely extra-axial in nature and the appearance is suggestive of a subdural empyema.

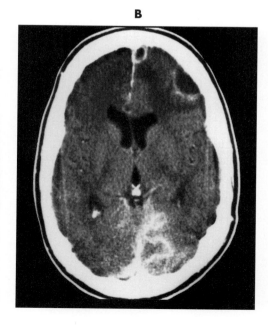

FIGURE 7-3, *B* (Contrast enhanced)

In addition to the empyema of the left frontal region, abnormal enhancement is identified posteriorly above the tentorium cerebelli. This represents spread of subdural empyema along the falx from its most anterior to posterior margin and from there over the top of the tentorium cerebelli.

Patient 7-4 • Herpes Simplex Encephalitis

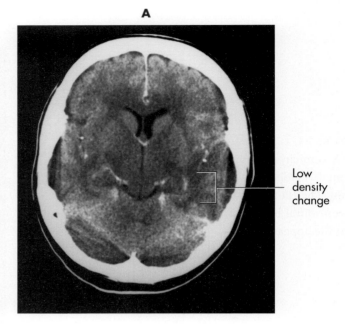

FIGURE 7-4, *A* (Contrast enhanced)

There is an area of low density change in the left temporal region, which, although subtle, is better delineated from the normal density and surrounding cortex than on the noncontrast CT (not included). There is subtle localized mass effect.

Low density change

B

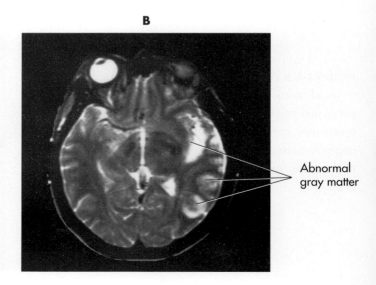

FIGURE 7-4, *B* (Noncontrast T2W MRI)

There is inhomogeneous hyperintense signal in the cortex of the left temporal lobe consistent with herpes simplex encephalitis given the clinical setting.

Abnormal gray matter

Patient 7-5 • Progressive Multifocal Leukoencephalopathy

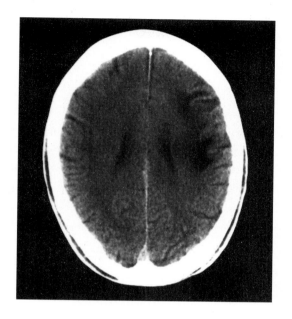

FIGURE 7-5 (Noncontrast)

There is an abnormal low density area in the subcortical white matter of the left frontal lobe. This extends into the white matter structures immediately beneath the overlying gray matter of the gyrus, particularly anteriorly. *This appearance is atypical for infarction because the gray matter is spared.* In the clinical setting of an immunocompromised patient, this is quite specific for progressive multifocal leukoencephalopathy (PML). This abnormality typically does not enhance.

Patient 7-6 • Toxoplasmosis

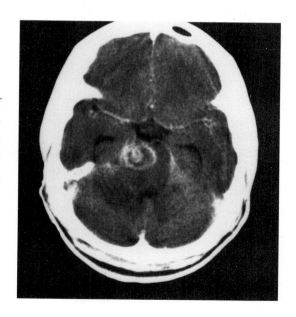

FIGURE 7-6 (Contrast enhanced)

A ring-enhancing lesion is seen in the right side of the midbrain with an associated central smaller enhancing ring lesion. The low density change in the surrounding brainstem and right middle cerebellar peduncle is consistent with accompanying edema. This patient was immunocompromised and this is presumed to represent toxoplasmosis in view of a favorable response to therapy.

Patient 7-7 • Cysticercosis

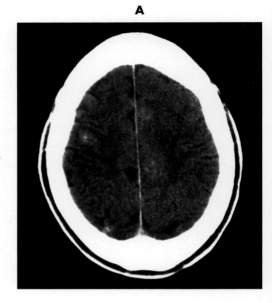

A

FIGURE 7-7, *A* (Noncontrast)

Three or four very subtle hyperdensities can be identified and some, particularly on the right, appear to have a focal central hyperdensity consistent with calcification.

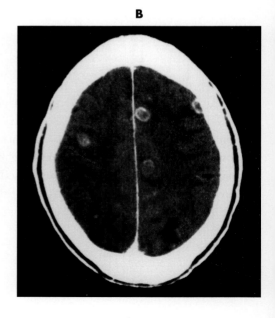

B

FIGURE 7-7, *B* (Contrast enhanced)

These subtle hyperdensities show significant enhancement, particularly peripherally in a ring-type fashion, and their central calcifications are more readily apparent. The appearance is most suggestive of neurocysticercosis.

CHAPTER 8

MISCELLANEOUS CONDITIONS

Hydrocephalus, atrophy, and various other important neurologic problems are arbitrarily grouped together in this chapter.

Hydrocephalus/Atrophy

The essentials of interpreting hydrocephalus and atrophy are explained in Chapter One. Multiple other examples in this atlas in which hydrocephalus is secondary to trauma, SAH, and neoplasms can be found in the chapters relating to these topics.

Patient 8-1 • Obstructive (Noncommunicating) Hydrocephalus

A

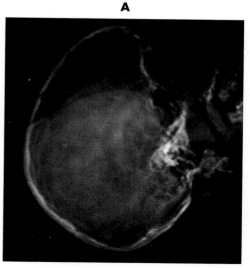

FIGURE 8-1, *A* (Scout view)

This demonstrates an abnormal architecture of the skull vault known as a "brass beaten skull." This finding is suggestive of long standing hydrocephalus. The increased intracranial pressure, which has occurred over a long period of time in this child, has remodeled the inner table of the skull into the form of multiple gyral indentations.

Continued

FIGURE 8-1, *B* (Noncontrast)

There is marked enlargement of the lateral and third ventricles. Hypodense change surrounding the frontal horns is suggestive of *transependymal CSF flow,* as is often seen in *acute* hydrocephalus. Transependymal CSF resorption is evident when there is frontal periventricular hypodensity associated with hydrocephalus. There is also suggestion of an isodense space occupying lesion near the outlet of the fourth ventricle that proved to represent a tectal glioma. The hydrocephalus of the lateral and third ventricles with a normal fourth ventricle (image not reproduced) implies obstruction at the level of the aqueduct.

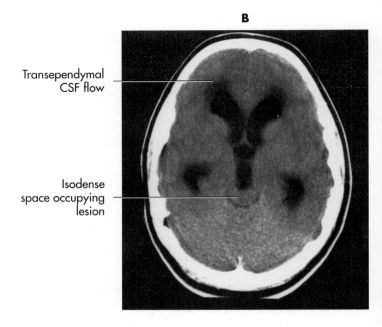

B

Transependymal CSF flow

Isodense space occupying lesion

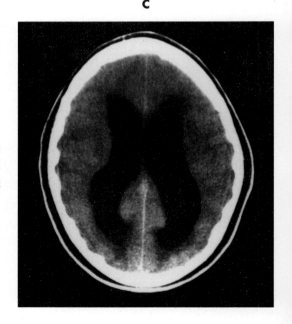

C

FIGURE 8-1, *C* (Noncontrast)

The marked hydrocephalus of the lateral ventricles is evident on this more superior cut. The corrugated appearance of the inner table of the skull is consistent with "brass beaten skull."

Patient 8-2 • Obstructive Hydrocephalus

FIGURE 8-2, A (Noncontrast)

This demonstrates marked dilatation of the lateral ventricles in the area of the frontal horns and the third ventricle. The third ventricle tapers toward the cerebral aqueduct. The appearance is suggestive of severe obstructive hydrocephalus, probably of a long standing nature that is presently *in a balanced state because there is no transependymal CSF resorption* in the area of the frontal horns. Transependymal CSF resorption is evident when there is frontal periventricular hypodensity associated with hydrocephalus (see Figure 8-1, *B* and *C*).

The hydrocephalus probably results from aqueductal stenosis.

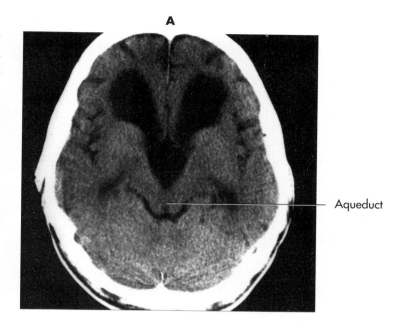

Aqueduct

FIGURE 8-2, B (Noncontrast)

On this more superior cut the marked hydrocephalus affecting the lateral ventricles is immediately apparent. There are relatively normal cortical sulci in keeping with severe hydrocephalus in a balanced state (see Figure 8-4, *B,* for effaced cortical sulci secondary to acute obstructive hydrocephalus).

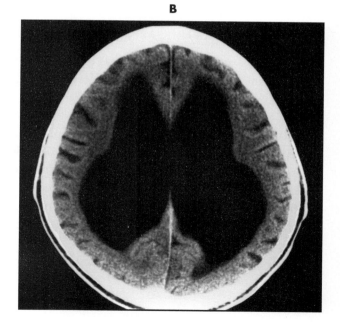

Patient 8-3 • Atrophy with Secondary Ventricular Enlargement

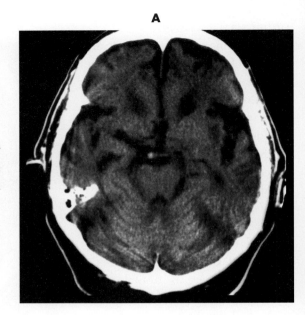

A

FIGURE 8-3, *A* (Noncontrast)

This demonstrates enlargement of the suprasellar cistern and both Sylvian fissures and atrophy of the cerebellum, suggesting a combination of cerebral and cerebellar atrophy.

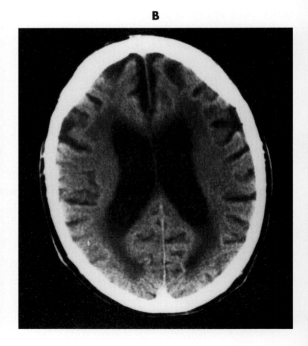

B

FIGURE 8-3, *B* (Noncontrast)

This shows ventricular enlargement in combination with enlargement of the cortical sulci diffusely. In addition there are patchy periventricular hypodensities. The combination of ventricular and sulcal enlargement is most in keeping with hydrocephalus on an ex vacuo basis secondary to diffuse cerebral atrophy. The more pronounced dilatation of the ventricles suggests that the atrophy is predominantly subcortical in nature. The patchy periventricular hypodensities are in keeping with a leukomalacia, which usually results from small vessel cerebral angiopathy, i.e., this is leukomalacia not transependymal flow.

Patient 8-4 • Shunt Dysfunction

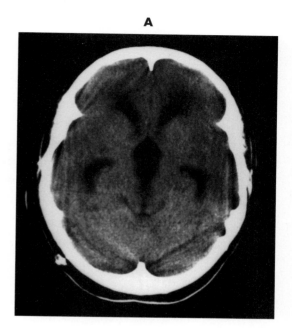

A

FIGURE 8-4, A (Noncontrast)

There is marked dilatation of the third ventricle with tapering at the level of the cerebral aqueduct and associated dilatation of the temporal horns. Transependymal flow of CSF is present.

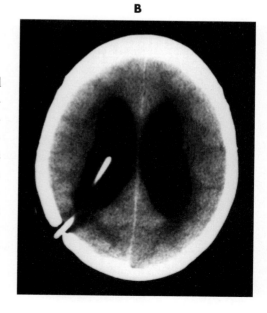

B

FIGURE 8-4, B (Noncontrast)

Marked hydrocephalus affects the lateral ventricles, and the *diffuse effacement of the cortical sulci is in keeping with severe active hydrocephalus* despite the presence of a right ventricular shunt catheter (see Figure 8-2, *B*, for hydrocephalus in a balanced state). Overall, the appearance is consistent with acute obstructive hydrocephalus at the level of the cerebral aqueduct causing dilatation of the lateral and third ventricles. Given the presence of a shunt catheter and a previously normal study one month before, these images are consistent with acute shunt dysfunction.

Patient 8-5 • Shunt Dysfunction

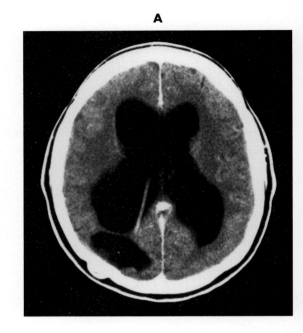

A

FIGURE 8-5 (Noncontrast)

This demonstrates marked hydrocephalus despite the presence of a right parietal shunt. There is also a well-defined hypodensity posterior to the right lateral ventricle consistent with a porencephalic cyst (see Chapter 9, p. 179). Given the fact that this is located in the area of the shunt this cyst probably resulted from a remote posterior cerebral artery infarction following shunt insertion.

Patient 8-6 • Atrophy with Enlargement of the Sulci, Cisterns, and Ventricles

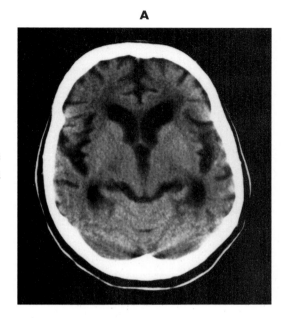

A

FIGURE 8-6, *A* (Noncontrast)

This is atrophy rather than hydrocephalus because there is enlargement of the lateral ventricles, the Sylvian fissures, and cortical sulci.

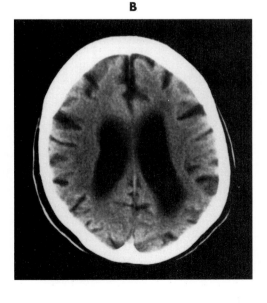

B

FIGURE 8-6, *B* (Noncontrast)

This image demonstrates more completely the lateral ventricular enlargement and the enlargement of the cortical sulci, which is somewhat inhomogeneous in distribution. The appearance remains consistent with moderate atrophy that may be slightly more prominent subcortically.

Patient 8-7 • Mild Atrophy

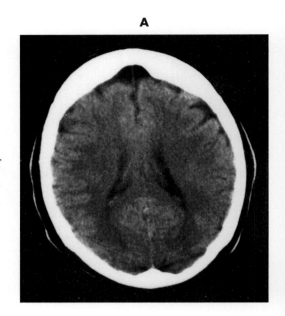

FIGURE 8-7, *A* (Noncontrast)

   The normal ventricular size but slight prominence of the cortical sulci in the frontal regions is suggestive of an early degree of predominantly cortical cerebral atrophy.

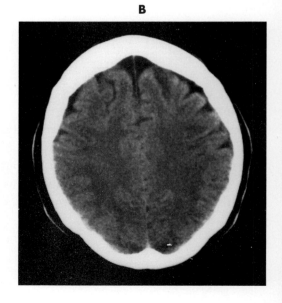

FIGURE 8-7, *B* (Noncontrast)

   This slice is one higher than the previous and again demonstrates slight prominence of the cortical sulci in the frontal regions, suggesting that early predominantly cortical cerebral atrophy may exist.

Other Miscellaneous Conditions

Patient 8-8 • **Diffuse Cerebral Anoxia Postcardiac Arrest**

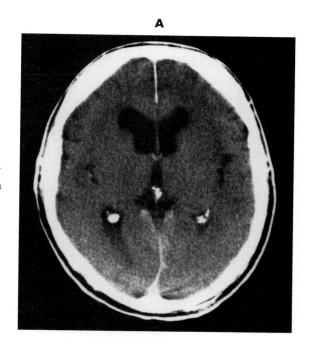

FIGURE 8-8, *A* (Noncontrast)

Diffuse loss of the gray-white matter differentiation at the cortical, subcortical and basal ganglia levels due to infarction of the gray matter.

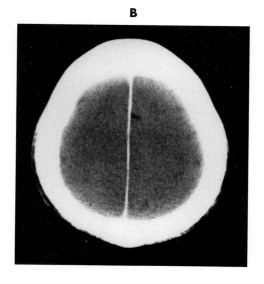

FIGURE 8-8, *B* (Noncontrast)

Complete loss of gray-white matter differentiation.

Patient 8-9 • Fat Droplets

FIGURE 8-9 (Noncontrast)

The multiple, tiny extreme hypodensities in the subarachnoid and intraventricular spaces are consistent with air or fat. The measurement of the actual attenuation co-efficients of these droplets was more in keeping with fat and this is consistent with the final diagnosis of ruptured dermoid cyst. The less profound hypodensity in the left basal ganglia is compatible with a nonacute lacunar type infarction.

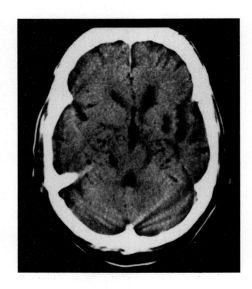

Patient 8-10 • Postradiation Leukomalacia

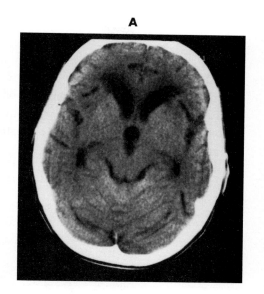

A

FIGURE 8-10, *A* (Noncontrast)

There are confluent hypodensities in the periventricular white matter adjacent to both frontal horns.

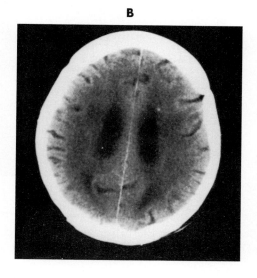

B

FIGURE 8-10, *B* (Noncontrast)

There are extensive periventricular and subcortical hypodensities. These are in keeping with extensive leukoencephalopathy. Their confluent nature is somewhat atypical for leukoencephalopathy secondary to angiopathy. These were due to cranial irradiation. Compare this image to a normal CT (Figure 1-9, *D* and *E*) to better appreciate these abnormal hypodensities.

Patient 8-11 • Central Pontine Myelinolysis

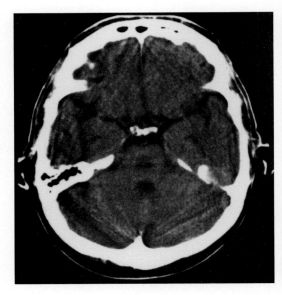

FIGURE 8-11 (Noncontrast)

Note the relatively well defined hypodensity in the central pontine location. Given a previous history of alcoholism and hyponatremia this is consistent with central pontine myelinolysis.

Patient 8-12 • Paget's Disease

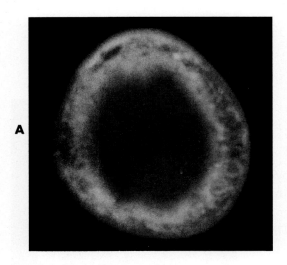

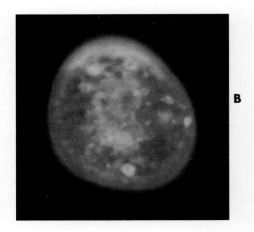

FIGURE 8-12, *A* (Bone window)

This bone window demonstrates marked thickening of the calvarium with altered areas of bony sclerosis and lysis consistent with a diagnosis of Paget's disease.

FIGURE 8-12, *B* (Bone window)

This slice obtained at the vertex nicely demonstrates the altered areas of bony lysis and sclerosis typical of Paget's disease.

Patient 8-13 • Intraparenchymal Calcification

FIGURE 8-13 (Noncontrast)

The well-circumscribed nodular hyperdensity in the left frontal lobe sub-cortically is likely a focus of dystrophic calcification. This is possibly in association with previous exposure to an infectious agent, perhaps granulomatous in nature. These are usually incidental findings in the absence of seizure disorder, in which case further investigation is warranted.

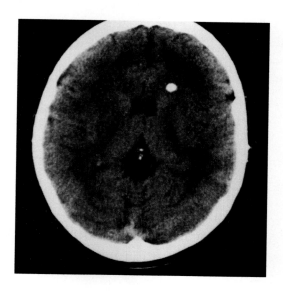

Patient 8-14 • Leukoencephalopathy (Leukomalacia) Probably from Binswanger's Disease

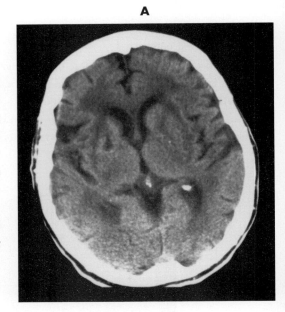

A

FIGURE 8-14, *A* (Noncontrast)

Extensive low density change in the periventricular white matter is most apparent around the frontal horns. These confluent hypodensities extend into the basal ganglia near the internal/external capsules. The appearance is consistent with leukoencephalopathy (leukomalacia). Given the advanced age and dementia of the patient, this is most likely due to subcortical arteriosclerotic encephalopathy (SAE), also called Binswanger's disease. The well-defined hypodensity in the right putamen is consistent with a nonacute lacunar type infarction.

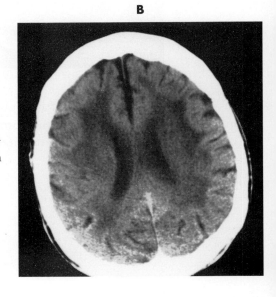

B

FIGURE 8-14, *B* (Noncontrast)

This cut higher up demonstrates extensive periventricular and subcortical hypodensities in keeping with an advanced leukoencephalopathy (leukomalacia).

Patient 8-15 • Leukoencephalopathy and Atrophy

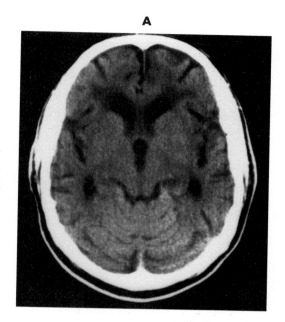

FIGURE 8-15, *A* (Noncontrast)

Mild to moderate prominence of the ventricular system in association with patchy periventricular hypodensities in the frontal region. This should not be termed SAE or Binswanger's disease in the absence of dementia.

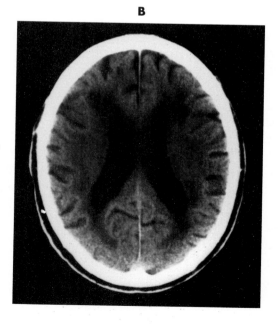

FIGURE 8-15, *B* (Noncontrast)

This demonstrates extensive patchy periventricular and subcortical hypodensities in association with moderate prominence of the ventricles and mild prominence of the cortical sulci. The pattern suggests moderate, predominantly subcortical cerebral atrophy in association with an extensive periventricular and subcortical leukoencephalopathy (leukomalacia).

Patient 8-16 • Arachnoid Cyst

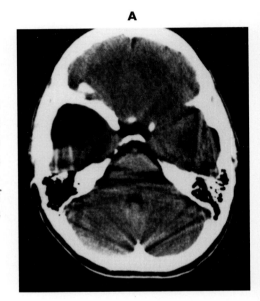

A

FIGURE 8-16, *A* (Noncontrast)

A well-defined hypodensity in the right middle cranial fossa abuts the sphenoid wing and displays a sharply defined posterior margin outlined by the right temporal lobe. This appearance is characteristic for a right middle cranial fossa arachnoid cyst. These cysts most commonly result from accumulation of CSF within developmental abnormalities of the meninges but may also occur secondary to adhesions from meningitis, SAH, and trauma.

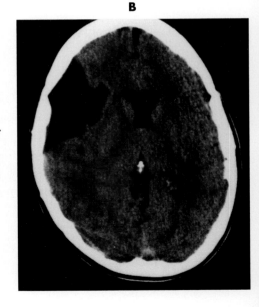

B

FIGURE 8-16, *B* (Noncontrast)

The well-defined arachnoid cyst extends to the level of the right Sylvian fissure. Associated with the cyst are: temporal lobe hypoplasia, some focal right frontal hypoplasia, and slight right sided mass effect.

Patient 8-17 • **Pseudotumor Cerebri**

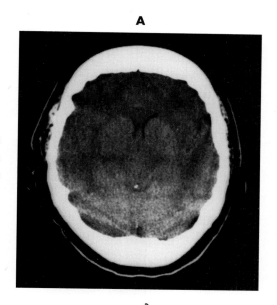

FIGURE 8-17, *A* (Noncontrast)

This demonstrates small frontal horns and diffuse effacement of the basal cisterns, as well as the Sylvian fissures bilaterally. In the appropriate clinical setting, this is in keeping with the diagnosis of pseudotumor cerebri.

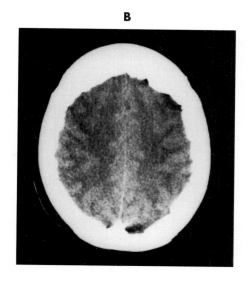

FIGURE 8-17, *B* (Noncontrast)

There is diffuse sulcal effacement. Compare this image with a normal CT at this level (Figure 1-8, *K*).

Patient 8-18 • Advanced Multiple Sclerosis

FIGURE 8-18, *A* (Noncontrast)

Patchy periventricular hypodensities are present bilaterally, particularly adjacent to the frontal horns and atria of both lateral ventricles. The normal vein of Galen is also seen (see Figure 9-1).

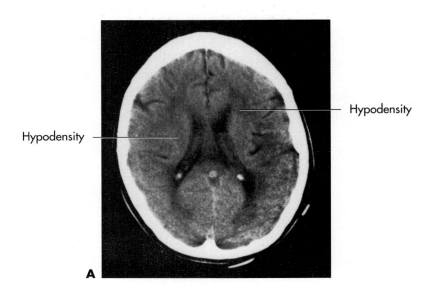

Hypodensity

Hypodensity

A

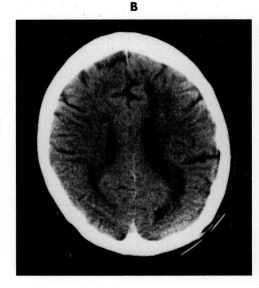

B

FIGURE 8-18, *B* (Noncontrast)

Confluent and more focal periventricular hypodensities, the latter seen more anteriorly. These represent areas of demyelination in a patient with extensive multiple sclerosis (MS). CT is usually normal in patients with milder MS and the emergency use of CT would be to rule out other causes of the patient's symptoms.

MRI is more sensitive for the lesions of MS.

Patient 8-19 • Tension Pneumocephalus

The sequence of images shows an abnormal intracranial collection that has the density of air. The brain is severely compressed. This neurosurgical emergency resulted after a vigorous sneeze in a patient with recent facial surgery and a disrupted cribiform plate.

Usually pneumocephalus has no mass effect. If mass effect is present, it implies that the air is accumulating under tension.

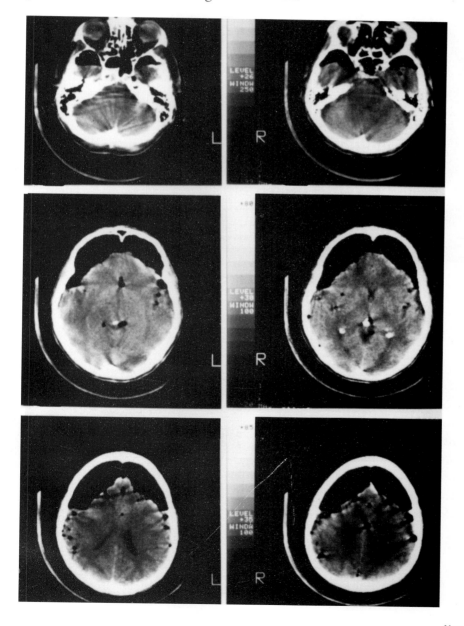

CHAPTER 9

VARIATIONS OF NORMAL STRUCTURES, ARTIFACTS, AND CONGENITAL ABNORMALITIES

Variations of Normal Structures

Occasionally, we are initially puzzled by seeing a structure that we do not recall seeing before but which gives us the impression of probably being normal. The images in this chapter are examples of such that have been brought to our attention recurrently by house staff and colleagues—the images represent normal vascular structures, calcifications, subarachnoid spaces and cisterns, and sulci that have a prominent or unusual appearance.

Examples of other variations of normal structures and artifacts are included throughout the book.

Artifacts

Motion Artifact

Patient motion has a devastating effect on image quality. The first type of motion artifact involves movement in which all elements of the CT slice remain in the beam throughout the exposure but the elements change orientation to each other. This produces black and white vertical bands for side-to-side motion and diagonal bands for rotary motion. An even more damaging type of artifact occurs when the elements move completely out of the beam portion of the exposure. This type of motion is most disruptive of image quality when high contrast objects such as bone or air move in or out of the beam.

Streak Artifact

Streak artifact is due to the major aberration that occurs at the interface between two different tissues with linear attenuation co-efficients that differ by greater than 60%. The computer reconstruction "undershoots" the density of soft tissues (brain, cerebral spinal fluid) at the junction with bone producing a lucent 2 to 6 mm area adjacent to the bone. This is an especially common artifact at the internal occipital protuberance. A similar phenomenon occurs at air/soft tissue interfaces, but with "overshoot" a ring of apparent greater density is seen within the soft tissues of the brain and cerebral spinal fluid.

Volume Averaging

The volume average and calculated linear attenuation co-efficient for a pixel is a weighted average of all materials in the pixel. Because the photoelectric attenuation is much greater for calcium than for cerebral spinal fluid, a small amount of calcium increases the average toward a higher linear attenuation co-efficient. Therefore even a small amount of calcium can make the entire picture element appear white. This effect is called partial volume averaging effect.

Finally, an apparent increase in skull thickness can occur when the skull is cut obliquely. This usually occurs in the more superficial cuts. This produces a shaded area in which the brain tissue is hidden from view by the calvarium.

Congenital Malformations

In the emergency setting most congenital malformations have little clinical relevance provided they are correctly interpreted. Most congenital malformations today are best classified and characterized using MR imaging.

CSF Containing Abnormalities

ARACHNOID CYST

One of the most common congenital malformations seen is that of the arachnoid cyst, which typically appears as a very well circumscribed hypodensity whose attenuation numbers are consistent with CSF content. Most typically these are located in the middle cranial fossa abutting the sphenoid wing and are typically associated with a degree of hypoplasia of the adjacent temporal lobe. Less common locations include the quadrigeminal plate and posterior fossa, the latter in the area of the cerebellopontine angle cistern. These less common arachnoid cysts may be associated with accompanying hydrocephalus if there is compression of the adjacent cerebral aqueduct or fourth ventricle.

VENTRICLES

Mild asymmetry of the lateral ventricles between the left and right sides is frequently observed as a normal variant. Nevertheless, in these cases one must always analyze the CT carefully, especially the adjacent cuts, to ensure that this asymmetry is not secondary to pathology.

Another frequent CSF-containing congenital abnormality can be seen in the midline in three basic locations, none of which usually have any clinical significance. These include a CSF collection between the septum pellucidum separating the frontal horns of both lateral ventricles, the so-called cavum septi pellucidi. If the CSF-containing collection extends posterior to the level of the foramina of Munro, an additional cavum vergae is present. If the CSF collection is above the roof of the third ventricle between the medial border of the atria of both lateral ventricles then the term *cavum velum interpositum* is used.

Abnormalities in the shape of the ventricular system can be seen secondary to underlying congenital malformations. An abnormal configuration of the lateral ventricles in which the frontal horns are hypoplastic and parallel and the occipital horns are enlarged is termed *colpocephaly* and is associated with agenesis or dysgenesis of the corpus callosum. A widened midline communication of the fourth ventricle with the cisterna magna is seen in association with a Dandy-Walker variant: if the cisterna magna is enlarged and there is hypoplasia or absence of the cerebellar hemispheres, a true Dandy-Walker malformation is present.

Porencephalic cysts: CSF-containing collections that are well circumscribed but surrounded by normal brain parenchyma are termed *porencephalic cysts* if they communicate with the ventricular system. They are termed *pseudoporencephalic cysts* if there is no apparent communication.

Schizencephaly: CSF-filled clefts in the cerebral hemispheres that extend from the cortical mantle to the level of the lateral ventricle but are continuously lined by gray matter and associated with correspondingly little white matter are termed *areas of schizencephaly*. These may be unilateral or bilateral and narrow or wide and are termed *closed* or *open lip schizencephaly* respectively. These patients often have contralateral body weakness in association with cerebral seizure disorder.

Hemispheres

Often a significant asymmetry exists between the two cerebral hemispheres. Usually this implies relative atrophy of the affected hemisphere. This manifests usually as enlargement of the ipsilateral lateral ventricle and cortical sulci. There may be compensatory changes in the ipsilateral skull to accommodate this long standing hemiatrophy in the form of a thickened skull vault and overdeveloped paranasal sinuses. This condition is termed *congenital hemiatrophy* and is often seen in association with weak extremities of the contralateral side of the body. There may or may not be an associated seizure disorder.

Vascular Structures

Prominent vein of Galen

Noteworthy Point: Always consider a diagnosis of thrombosis of the deep venous system if the vein of Galen appears large or abnormally dense. Associated findings on CT that may be present with deep venous thrombosis are: (1) increased density of adjacent venous structures such as the straight sinus or internal cerebral veins or (2) hypodensity of the basal ganglia, especially the thalami, which may represent venous infarcts. See Figures 3-16 to 3-18 for true venous thrombosis.

Patient 9-1 • **Prominent Venous Structures**

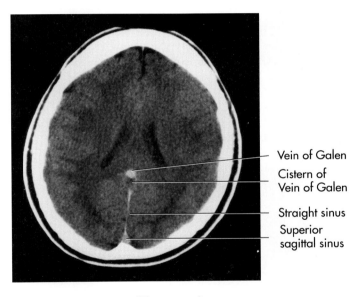

Vein of Galen
Cistern of
Vein of Galen

Straight sinus
Superior
sagittal sinus

FIGURE 9-1 (Noncontrast)

Patient 9-2 • **Prominent Vein of Galen**

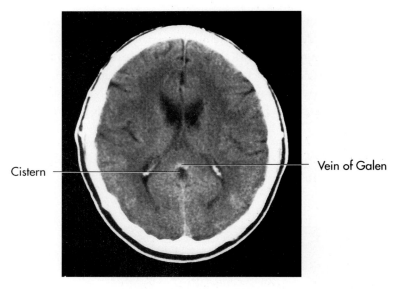

Cistern — — Vein of Galen

FIGURE 9-2 (Noncontrast)

Patient 9-3 • **Prominent Vein of Galen**

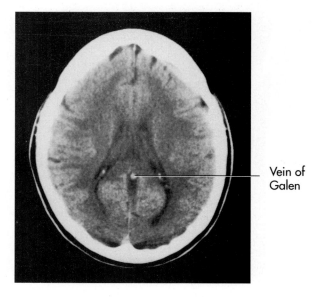

Vein of
Galen

FIGURE 9-3 (Noncontrast)

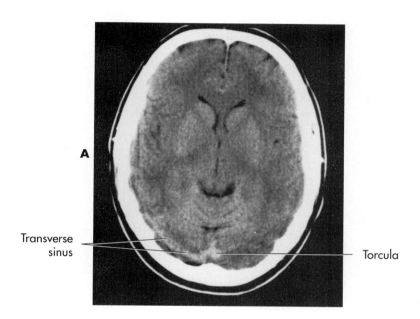

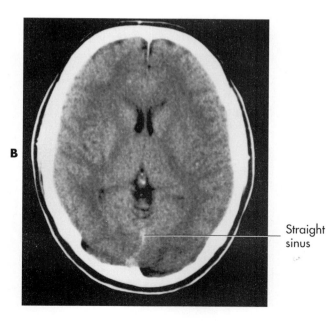

FIGURE 9-4, *A* **and** *B* (Noncontrast)

Patient 9-5 • Well-visualized Torcula (Venous Confluence) and Sagittal Sinus

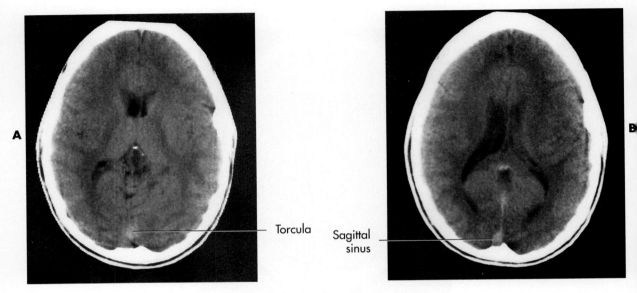

Torcula

Sagittal sinus

FIGURE 9-5, *A* and *B* (Noncontrast)

Patient 9-6 • Normal Basilar Artery and Tentorium

FIGURE 9-6 (Noncontrast)

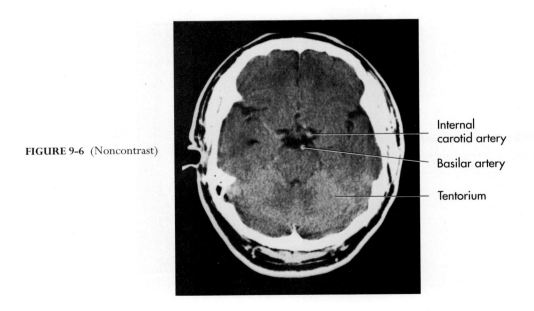

Internal carotid artery

Basilar artery

Tentorium

Calcifications

NOTE: Also see Figures 9-19 and 3-3 for calcification of the basal ganglia.

Patient 9-7 • Ossification or Calcification of the Falx

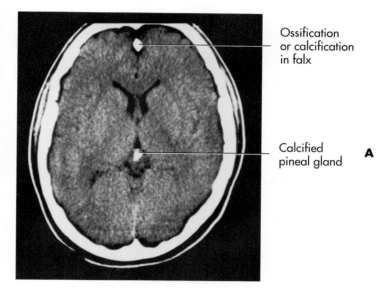

Ossification or calcification in falx

Calcified pineal gland

A

FIGURE 9-7, *A* (Noncontrast)

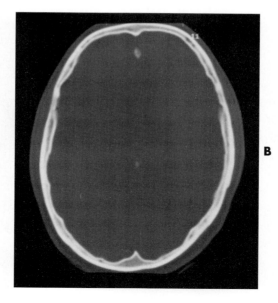

B

FIGURE 9-7, *B* (Bone window)
Calcified structures from Figure 9-7, *A*, as seen on bone window.

Patient 9-8 • Calcified Choroid Plexus (Bilateral)

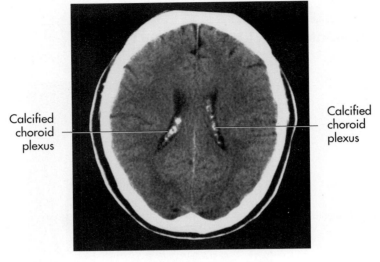

Calcified
choroid
plexus

Calcified
choroid
plexus

FIGURE 9-8 (Noncontrast)

Patient 9-9 • Calcified Choroid Plexus and Vertebral Artery Atheromata (Bilateral)

A

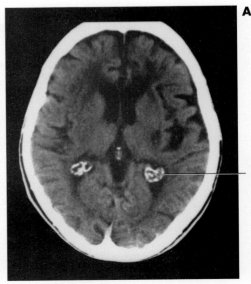

FIGURE 9-9, *A* (Noncontrast)

There is periventricular leukomalacia and a lacunar infarct in the left lentiform nucleus, as well as the benign calcifications.

Calcified
choroid
plexus

B

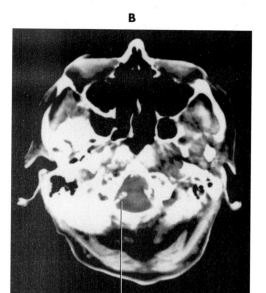

FIGURE 9-9, *B* (Bone window)

Calcified vertebral a. atheroma

Patient 9-10 • Calcified Choroid Plexus

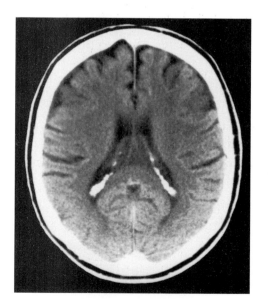

FIGURE 9-10 (Noncontrast)

Subarachnoid Spaces and Cisterns

Patient 9-11 • **Prominent Cisterna Magna
and Venous Confluence (Torcula)**

FIGURE 9-11, *A, B,* and *C* (Noncontrast)

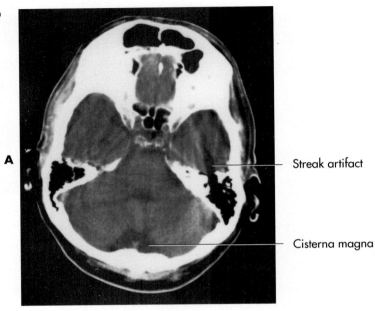

Streak artifact

Cisterna magna

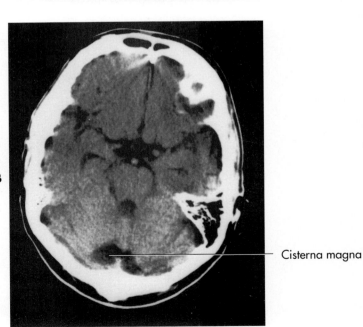

Cisterna magna

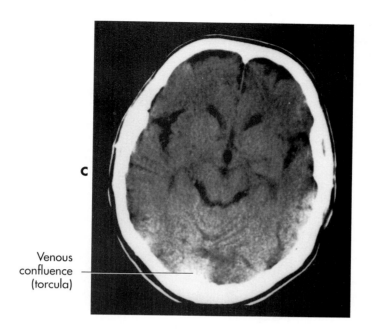

Venous
confluence
(torcula)

Patient 9-12 • **Prominent Superior Cerebellar Cistern (also see Figure 2-7)**

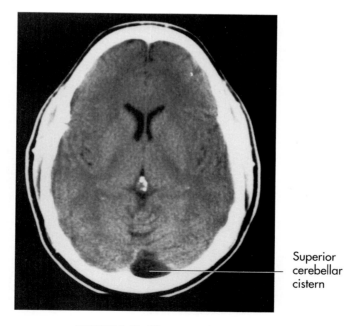

Superior
cerebellar
cistern

FIGURE 9-12 (Noncontrast)

Patient 9-13 • Superior Cerebellar Cistern, not to be Confused with
an Occipital Lobe Infarction

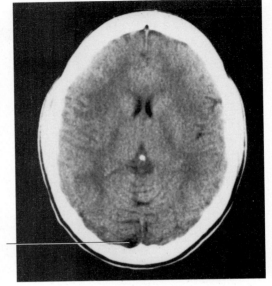

FIGURE 9-13 (Noncontrast)

Superior
cerebellar
cistern

Patient 9-14 • Junction of Ambient and Cerebropontine Angle Cistern (Bilateral)

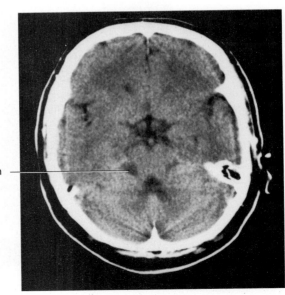

FIGURE 9-14 (Noncontrast)

Cistern

Patient 9-15 • Sulcal Prominence

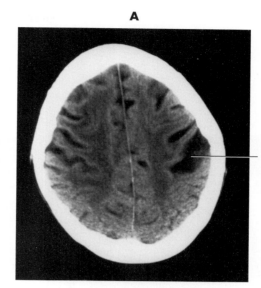

A

Prominent
central sulcus

FIGURE 9-15, *A* (Noncontrast)

There is a prominent central sulcus bilaterally, which is usually of little clinical significance. Mild atrophy is also present.

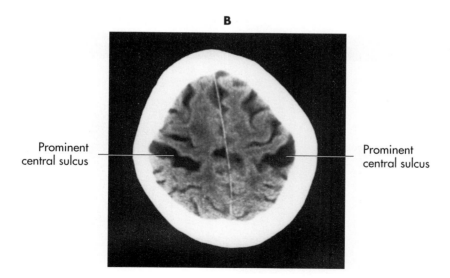

B

Prominent
central sulcus

Prominent
central sulcus

FIGURE 9-15, *B* (Noncontrast)

Miscellaneous

Patient 9-16 • Variants of Ventricles: Cavum Septi Pellucidi

This is a relatively common developmental variation of the ventricles.

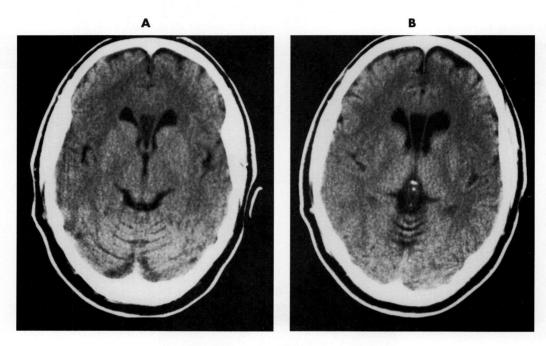

FIGURE 9-16, *A* **and** *B* (Noncontrast)

Patient 9-17 • (1) Variants of Ventricles: Cavum Septi Pellucidi and Cavum Vergae, (2) Calcification Choroid Plexus

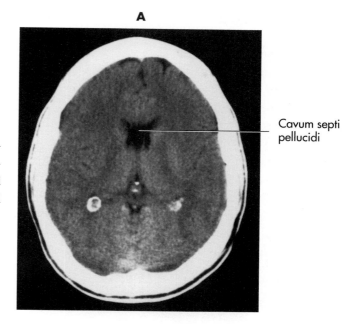

A

Cavum septi pellucidi

FIGURE 9-17, *A* (Noncontrast)

This demonstrates CSF density between the leaves of the septum pellucidum consistent with a cavum septi pellucidi located medial to both frontal horns.

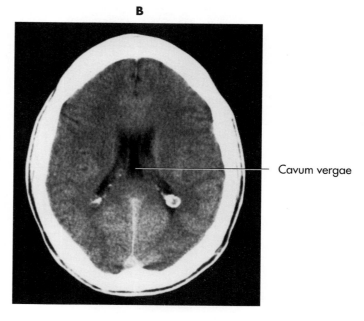

B

Cavum vergae

FIGURE 9-17, *B* (Noncontrast)

This slice, obtained 10 mm higher than the previous, demonstrates the cavum septum pellucidum in continuity with a cavum vergae. The cavum vergae is also of CSF density but is located more posterior than the cavum septum pelucidi. The tiny hyperdensity in the body of the right lateral ventricle anterior to the choroid glomus is calcification in the most anterior portion of the choroid plexus of the right lateral ventricle.

Patient 9-18 • **Petrous Bone Beam Hardening Artifact**

FIGURE 9-18 (Noncontrast)

"Beam hardening" refers to the filtration of lower energy x-ray photons when the beam crosses a thick section of bone, i.e., both petrous bones. The detectors receive more high energy photons emitted from the x-ray source and the computer reconstruction process then assumes that the soft tissue transversed by the x-ray was of a lower density. This accounts for the apparent hypodense area around the pons. The pons itself *appears* hyperdense relative to this low density and the computer and the eye are tricked into thinking that the pons is hyperdense.

This artifact should not be confused with hemorrhage in the pons. This patient presented with acute headache and had a normal neurologic examination, which would not be consistent with pontine hemorrhage.

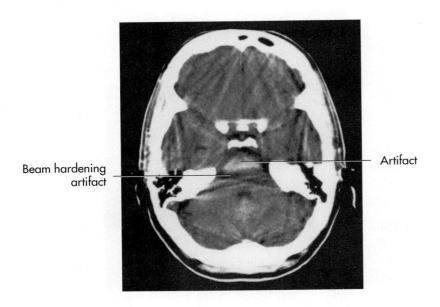

Beam hardening artifact

Artifact

Patient 9-19 • Plagiocephaly (Crooked Skull) and Mild Cortical Atrophy with Prominent Subarachnoid Space

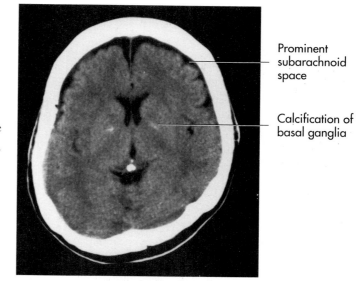

Prominent subarachnoid space

Calcification of basal ganglia

FIGURE 9-19 (Noncontrast)

Plagiocephaly is caused by premature unilateral closure of a suture. In this case, probably the left side of the lambdoid.

Patient 9-20 • Cavum Velum Interpositum

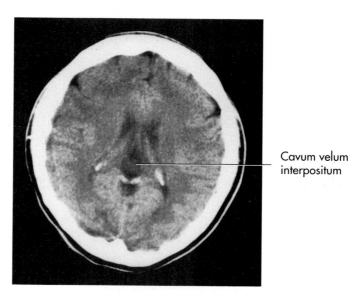

Cavum velum interpositum

FIGURE 9-20 (Noncontrast)

The round hypodensity in the mid line is a CSF filled developmental variant located above the third ventricle and below the corpus callosum.

INDEX

A

Abnormalities
    cerebrospinal fluid containing, 178-179
    congenital, variations of normal structures and artifacts and, 177-195
Abscess(es), 150, 151, 152
    cerebral, 150, 151, 152
        gas collections caused by, 8
    contrast enhancing, 4
Acoustic neurinoma, 118, 124
    CT characteristics of, 120
Active hydrocephalus, 6
Acute epidural hematoma
    classic, 32
    in middle cranial fossa, 36
Acute frontal intracerebral clot, 93
Acute hemorrhage, 7
    in intrahemispheric fissure, bifrontal contusions and, 54
Acute intracerebral hemorrhage, 106
Acute on chronic subdural hematoma, 45
    with fluid/fluid level, 50
Acute subarachnoid hemorrhage, 91, 92, 93
    in basal cisterns, 5
Acute subdural hematoma; see Subdural hematoma, acute
Adenoma, pituitary, 125
    CT characteristics of, 120
Adult
    middle-aged, normal brain anatomy of, noncontrast, 23-26
    young, normal brain anatomy of
        contrast-enhanced, 26-28
        noncontrast, 16-22
Advanced multiple sclerosis, 174
Agenesis of corpus callosum, 179
Air
    hypodensities caused by, 7-8
    intracranial, occipital acute subdural hematoma with, 42
    in scalp hematoma, 60-61
Air cells
    ethmoid, in normal young adult, 21, 22
    mastoid
        basal skull fracture through, 60-61
        in normal young adult, 16, 21
Ambient cisterns
    and cerebropontine angle cistern, junction of, variation in, 190
    compression of, 46

Ambient cisterns, *cont'd*
    in middle-aged adult, 23
    in normal young adult, 10, 18
Anatomy, CT, normal, 9-29
    variations in, 177-195
Aneurysm(s)
    anterior communicating artery, nontraumatic hemorrhage caused by, 104
    atherosclerotic, fusiform, of basilar artery, 98
    cerebral, nontraumatic hemorrhage caused by, 103-104
    communicating artery, 97
    giant, 99, 100
    images of, 97-101
    middle cerebral artery, 94, 95, 98, 101
        nontraumatic hemorrhage caused by, 104
        subarachnoid hemorrhage caused by, 94
    mycotic, 150
    rupture of, 85
    subarachnoid hemorrhage and, 85-101
    suprasellar, 118
Aneurysmal sac, contrast enhancing, 4
Angioma(angiomata)
    cavernous, 113
        nontraumatic hemorrhage caused by, 104-105
    venous, 114
        nontraumatic hemorrhage caused by, 105
Anoxia, cerebral, diffuse, after cardiac arrest, 165
Anterior cerebral artery, 15
    herniation of, 49
    in normal young adult, 26
Anterior cerebral artery territory infarct, 73, 74-75
Anterior clinoid process, in normal young adult, 22
Anterior communicating artery, 15
    aneurysm of, nontraumatic hemorrhage caused by, 104
Anterior cranial fossa, in normal young adult, 22
Aqueduct
    cerebral, in middle-aged adult, 23
    in normal young adult, 18
    of Sylvius, metastatic small cell carcinoma of lung with obstruction of, 147-148
Aqueductal stenosis, congenital, 118
Arachnoid cyst(s), 118, 172
    causes of, 172
    congenital, 178-179

Arrest, cardiac; *see* Cardiac arrest
Arrested hydrocephalus, 6
Arteriosclerotic encephalopathy, subcortical, 170
Arteriovenous malformation, 110-111, 112
    contrast enhancing, 4
    nontraumatic hemorrhage caused by, 104
    subarachnoid hemorrhage caused by, 86
Artery(ies)
    basilar, 15
        fusiform atherosclerotic aneurysm of, 98
        in normal young adult, 17
        variations of, 184
    carotid, internal, 15
        in middle-aged adult, 23
    cerebellar, 15
    cerebral; *see* Cerebral artery(ies)
    communicating, 15
        aneurysm of, 97
        anterior, aneurysm of, nontraumatic hemorrhage caused by, 104
    normal anatomy of, 15
    pericallosal, in normal young adult, 27
    vertebral, 15
        atheroma of, 186-187
        in normal young adult, 26
Artifact(s)
    motion, 177
    petrous bone beam hardening, 194
    streak, 177
        from internal occipital protuberance, 41
    variations of normal structures and congenital abnormalities
        and, 177-195
Astrocytoma(s), 116-117, 133-138; *see also* Glioma(s)
    cerebellar, 132
        CT characteristics of, 120
    cystic, differentiation of, from intraventricular tumors, 116
Asymmetry
    hemispheric, 180
    ventricular, 179
Atheroma, vertebral artery, 186-187
Atherosclerotic aneurysm of basilar artery, fusiform, 98
Atrophy, 6
    cerebral, 163
    cortical, mild, plagiocephaly and, with prominent subarachnoid
        space, 195
    with enlargement of sulci and cisterns, 163
    hydrocephalus and, images showing, 157-164
    leukoencephalopathy (leukomalacia) and, 171
    mild, 164, 195
    with ventricular enlargement, 160, 163
Auditory canal in normal young adult
    external, 17, 22
    internal, 22
Averaging, volume, 177
Axial imaging, 2
Axonal injury, diffuse, occipital fracture and contrecoup punctate hemor-
    rhage and, 52-53

B

Bacterial infections, 149-150
Bacterial meningitis, 150
"Bag of worms" appearance with arteriovenous malformation, 104
Balanced hydrocephalus, 6
Basal cisterns
    axial view of, 11, 12
    CT scan analysis and, 5
    lateral view of, 10, 13
    normal anatomy of, 9-13
    subarachnoid hemorrhage of, 90
Basal skull fracture through mastoid air cells, 60-61
Basilar artery, 15
    fusiform atherosclerotic aneurysm of, 98
    in normal young adult, 17
    variations of, 184
Basilar artery territory infarction, 78-79
Basilar skull fracture, air collection caused by, 8
"Beam hardening," 194
Beam hardening artifact, petrous bone, 194
Berry aneurysm, rupture of, 85
Bifrontal contusions and acute hemorrhage in intrahemispheric fissure, 54
Bilateral watershed infarctions, 65
Binswanger's disease, leukoencephalopathy (leukomalacia) from, 170
Bone
    frontal, in normal young adult, 22
    petrous, beam hardening artifact of, 194
Brain
    abscess of, 150, 151, 152; *see also* Abscess(es)
    atrophy of; *see* Atrophy
    miscellaneous conditions involving, 157-175
        images showing, 165-175
    normal anatomy of
        in middle-aged adult, noncontrast, 23-26
        in young adult
            contrast-enhanced, 26-28
            noncontrast, 16-22
Brainstem infarction, 80-81
"Brass/beaten skull," 157, 158
Brightness, adjusting, 3
Bronchoalveolar carcinoma, metastatic, 143-144

C

Calcification(s), 7, 185-187
    of choroid plexus, 186-187, 193
    of falx, 185
        in normal young adult, 21
    infections causing, 149
    intraparenchymal, 169
Capillary telangiectasias, nontraumatic hemorrhage caused by, 105
Capsule, internal and external, in normal young adult, 19
Carcinoma
    bronchoalveolar, metastatic, 143-144
    differentiation of, from supratentorial intraventricular tumors, 116
    small cell, metastatic, of lung, 142, 146
        with obstruction of aqueduct of Sylvius, 147-148
    squamous cell, 119

Carcinomatosis, meningeal, 116
Cardiac arrest
    diffuse cerebral anoxia after, 165
    watershed infarctions with, 65
Carotid artery, internal, 15
    in middle-aged adult, 23
Carotid canal in normal young adult, 21
Caudate nucleus in normal young adult, 19
Cavernous angioma, 113
    nontraumatic hemorrhage caused by, 104-105
Cavernous sinus, 13, 14
Cavum septi pellucidi, 179, 192, 193
Cavum velum interpositum, 179, 195
Cavum vergae, 179, 193
Cells, air
    ethmoid, in normal young adult, 21, 22
    mastoid
        basal skull fracture through, 60-61
        in normal young adult, 16, 21
Central pontine myelinolysis, 168
Central sulcus in normal young adult, 21
Centrum semiovale in normal young adult, 20
Cerebellar artery, 15
Cerebellar astrocytoma, 132
    CT characteristics of, 120
Cerebellar atrophy with ventricular enlargement, 160; see also Atrophy
Cerebellar cistern, superior
    differentiating, from occipital lobe infarction, 190
    prominent, 189
Cerebellar cystic astrocytoma, differentiation of, from intraventricular
        tumors, 116
Cerebellar hemisphere infarction, 80
Cerebellar hemorrhage, 107, 108
Cerebellar peduncle, middle, in normal young adult, 18
Cerebellar tonsil in normal young adult, 17
Cerebellopontine angle tumors, 118, 123
Cerebellum
    in middle-aged adult, 23
    in normal young adult, 18
Cerebral abscess(es), 150, 151, 152
    gas collections caused by, 8
Cerebral aneurysm, nontraumatic hemorrhage caused by, 103-104
Cerebral anoxia, diffuse, after cardiac arrest, 165
Cerebral aqueduct in middle-aged adult, 23
Cerebral artery(ies), 15
    anterior
        herniation of, 49
        infarct around, 73, 74-75
    middle; see Middle cerebral artery
    in normal young adult, 26
    posterior, infarct around, 78
    watershed infarctions and, 65
Cerebral artery sign, hyperdense middle, 66-69
Cerebral atrophy, 6, 163; see also Atrophy
    with ventricular enlargement, 160
Cerebral contusions, trauma causing, 31

Cerebral edema
    diffuse, 5
        acute subdural hematoma and, 58-59
    mass effect with, 5
Cerebral infarction, 6-7, 63-84
    gray matter hypodensities caused by, 8
Cerebral metastases, 119
Cerebral vein(s)
    of Galen, great, 13; see also Vein(s) of Galen
    internal, in normal young adult, 27, 28
    major, 14
Cerebritis, 149-150
Cerebropontine angle and ambient cistern, junction of, variation in, 190
Cerebrospinal fluid
    abnormalities containing, 178-179
    obstruction of, 5
    route of flow of, 5-6
    transependymal flow of, 6
        in hydrocephalus, 158
Cerebrospinal fluid spaces, normal anatomy of, 9-13
Cervical fractures, trauma causing, 31
Chemical meningitis, 8
Chiasm, optic, in normal young adult, 18
Choroid plexus
    calcification of, 186-187, 193
    in middle-aged adult, 24
    in normal young adult, 19, 27
    papillomas of, differentiation of, from supratentorial intraventricular
        tumors, 116
Chronic infections, 149
Chronic subdural hematoma; see Subdural hematoma, chronic
Circle of Willis, 15
Cistern(s)
    ambient; see Ambient cisterns
    basal; see Basal cisterns
    cerebellar, superior
        differentiating, from occipital lobe infarction, 190
        prominent, 189
    enlargement of, atrophy with, 163
    of great cerebral vein of Galen, 10
    prepontine, in normal young adult, 18
    quadrigeminal plate, in normal young adult, 19
    suprasellar, in normal young adult, 18
    Sylvian, in middle-aged adult, 23
    variations of, 188-191
Cisterna magna, 10
    prominent, 188-189
Clinoid process, anterior, in normal young adult, 22
Clivus in normal young adult, 16, 21
Closed schizencephaly, 179
Clot, intracerebral, frontal, acute, 93
Colliculi
    in middle-aged adult, 23
    in normal young adult, 19
Colloid cyst(s), 128-130
    classic, 128
    differentiation of, from supratentorial intraventricular tumors, 116

Colloid cyst(s), *cont'd*
  intraventricular, CT characteristics of, 120
  of third ventricle, 118
Colpocephaly, 179
Communicating arteries, 15
  aneurysm of, 97
    anterior, nontraumatic hemorrhage caused by, 104
Communicating hydrocephalus, 5
  subarachnoid hemorrhage with, 85-86
Compression
  subarachnoid space, mass effect with, 5
  sulcal, 6-7
    in MCA territory infarct, 71
  ventricular, mass effect with, 5
Computed tomography (CT); *see also* CT scans
  disadvantages of, 2
  history of 1
  indications for, 1
  MRI versus, 1-2
  patient positioning for, 2
  physics of, 2-3
  tissue appearance on, 3
  window and level settings for, 3
Congenital abnormalities, variations of normal structures and artifacts and, 177-195
Congenital aqueductal stenosis, 118
Congenital hemiatrophy, 180
Congenital malformations, 178-180
Contrast medium, hyperdensity with, 7
Contrast versus noncontrast cranial CT scans, 4
Contrecoup punctate hemorrhage, occipital fracture and, and diffuse axonal injury, 52-53
Contusion(s)
  acute subdural hematoma with evolution of, 62
  bifrontal, and acute hemorrhage in intrahemispheric fissure, 54
  cerebral, trauma causing, 31
  frontal, 54, 62
  frontal skull fracture and, 55
  hemorrhagic, focal, 57
  parietal, 60-61
  punctate, trauma causing, 52-62
Corpus callosum, agenesis or dysgenesis of, 179
Cortical atrophy, 6
  mild, plagiocephaly and, with prominent subarachnoid space, 195
Cranial CT scans, contrast versus noncontrast, 4
Cranial fossa
  anterior, in normal young adult, 22
  arachnoid cyst of, 172
  middle
    acute epidural hematoma in, 36
    in normal young adult, 21, 22
Craniopharyngioma, 117
Crooked skull and cortical atrophy with prominent subarachnoid space, 195
CT scan(s); *see also* Computed tomography (CT)
  analysis of, 4-9
  contrast versus noncontrast, 4

CT scan(s), *cont'd*
  essentials of, 1-29
  "fogging" on, 64
  interpreting, checklist for, 29
  normal anatomy on, 9-29
    subarachnoid hemorrhage differentiated from, 95
  tumor characteristics on, 119, 120
CT scanner, 1
Cyst(s)
  arachnoid, 118, 172
    causes of, 172
    congenital, 178-179
  colloid; *see* Colloid cyst(s)
  dermoid, ruptured, 166
  porencephalic, 179
  pseudoporencephalic, 179
Cystic astrocytoma, cerebellar, differentiation of, from intraventricular tumors, 116
Cysticercosis, 156
Cytomegalovirus, 149

D

Dandy-Walker malformation, 179
Delta sign, 82
Density, tissue
  abnormalities in, 7-9
  changing, 3
Depressed skull fracture, 60-61
Dermoid cyst, ruptured, 166
Dermoids, fat hypodensities caused by, 8
Diffuse axonal injury, occipital fracture and contrecoup punctate hemorrhage and, 52-53
Diffuse cerebral anoxia after cardiac arrest, 165
Diffuse cerebral edema, 5
  acute subdural hematoma and, 58-59
Dilated temporal horns, 97
Disease
  Binswanger's, leukoencephalopathy (leukomalacia) from, 170
  Paget's, 168
Dorsum sellae in normal young adult, 16, 18
Dural malformation, subarachnoid hemorrhage caused by, 86
Dural sinus, venous thrombosis of, 83
Dysgenesis of corpus callosum, 179

E

Ear in normal young adult
  middle, 22
  pinna of, 16
Edema
  cerebral
    diffuse, 5
      acute subdural hematoma and, 58-59
    mass effect with, 5
  white matter, white matter hypodensities caused by, 8
Effacement; *see* Compression
Empyema, subdural, 150, 153

Encephalitis
    contrast obscuring, 4
    herpes simplex, 151, 154
Encephalomalacia, 64
    hypodensities caused by, 8
Encephalopathy, arteriosclerotic, subcortical, 170
Enlargement
    of sulci, cisterns, and ventricles, atrophy with, 163
    ventricular, atrophy with, 160, 163
Ependymoma(s), 117, 131
    CT characteristics of, 120
    differentiation of
        from cerebellar astrocytoma, 132
        from intraventricular tumors, 116
Epidermoid, cerebellopontine angle, 118
Epidural hematoma(s)
    acute
        classic, 32
        in middle cranial fossa, 36
    density changes with, 33
    differential diagnosis of, 35, 36
    large, 32
    midline and, 33
    occipital, 35
    skull fracture causing, 33
    subtle, 34
    suture lines and, 33, 37
    trauma causing, 31, 32-36
Ethmoid air cells in normal young adult, 21, 22
External auditory canal in normal young adult, 17, 22
External capsule in normal young adult, 19
Extra-axial metastases, 125-126
    CT characteristics of, 120
Extra-axial tumors, 116
    CT characteristics of, 120
    images showing, 121-132

F

Face, fractures of, trauma causing, 31
Falx cerebri
    calcification, in normal young adult, 21
    in middle-aged adult, 25
    in normal young adult, 20, 21
    ossification or calcification of, 185
    posterior, chronic and acute subdural hematoma and, 46-47
Fat, hypodensities caused by, 8, 166
Fat droplets, 166
Fissure
    interhemispheric
        acute subdural hematoma in, 43
        bifrontal contusions and acute hemorrhage in, 54
        in middle-aged adult, 24
        subarachnoid hemorrhage of, 89, 90
    Sylvian
        in middle-aged adult, 23
        in normal young adult, 18
        subarachnoid hemorrhage of, 87, 88, 89, 90, 91, 93, 94

Focal hemorrhage, 56
Focal hemorrhagic contusions, 57
Foramen magnum in normal young adult, 16, 21, 22
Foramen ovale in normal young adult, 21
Fossa
    cranial
        anterior, in normal young adult, 22
        arachnoid cyst of, 172
        middle
            acute epidural hematoma in, 36
            in normal young adult, 21, 22
    jugular, in normal young adult, 22
    pituitary, in normal young adult, 16
    posterior
        acute subdural hematoma in, 39
        hemorrhage in, 107, 108
Fourth ventricle
    in middle-aged adult, 23
    in normal young adult, 17, 18
    subarachnoid hemorrhage of, 91
    tumors of, 116
        differential diagnosis of, 116
Fracture(s)
    air collections caused by, 8
    cervical, trauma causing, 31
    facial, trauma causing, 31
    occipital, and contrecoup punctate hemorrhage and diffuse axonal
        injury, 52-53
    skull; see Skull fracture(s)
Frontal bone in normal young adult, 22
Frontal contusion, 54, 62
Frontal horn in normal young adult, 18
Frontal hypoplasia, 172
Frontal intracerebral clot, acute, 93
Frontal lobe
    in normal young adult, 17, 21
    subarachnoid hemorrhage of, 91
Frontal region, acute subdural hematoma near, 37
Frontal sinus in normal young adult, 16, 21, 22
Frontal skull fracture, contusion and, 55
Fusiform atherosclerotic aneurysm of basilar artery, 98

G

Galen, vein of, 13
    in middle-aged adult, 24
    in normal young adult, 20
    prominent, 181, 182
    venous thrombosis of, 81
Ganglioglioma, 117
Gantry, 2
Gas, hypodensities caused by, 7-8
Giant aneurysm, 99, 100
Gland, pineal, in normal young adult, 19
Glioblastoma multiforme, 117, 135, 136, 137
Glioma(s), 116-117, 133-138
    high grade, versus lymphoma, 138
    of hypothalamus, 117-118

Glioma(s), *cont'd*
  intra-axial, CT characteristics of, 120
  lack of contrast enhancement of, 9
  low grade, 133, 134
  of optic chiasm, 117
  tectal, 118
Gliomatosis cerebri, 117
Globe in normal young adult, 16
Gray matter hypodensities, 8
Gray-white interface, loss of differentiation of, 8
  in diffuse cerebral anoxia postcardiac arrest, 165
  from infarction, 63, 71
Great cerebral vein of Galen, 13; *see also* Vein(s) of Galen
Gyrus, precentral, in normal young adult, 21

H

"Hardening, beam," 194
Head
  CT scans of; *see also* CT scans
    essentials of, 1-29
    interpreting, checklist for, 29
  images showing, 165-175
  miscellaneous conditions involving, 157-175
Headache, acute, 85
Hemangioblastoma, 140-141
  CT characteristics of, 120
Hematocrit effect, 50
Hematoma(s)
  epidural; *see* Epidural hematoma
  scalp, air in, 60-61
  subdural; *see* Subdural hematoma
Hemiatrophy, congenital, 180
Hemispheres
  asymmetry of, 180
  congenital malformations of, 180
Hemorrhage(s)
  acute, 7
    in intrahemispheric fissure, bifrontal contusions and, 54
    trauma causing, 31
  cerebellar, 107, 108
  focal, 56
  intracerebral, 105
    acute, 106
    contrast obscuring, 4
  intracranial, 94
  intraparenchymal
    and intraventricular, 107
    subarachnoid hemorrhage with, 85
  intraventricular
    and intraparenchymal, 107
    subarachnoid hemorrhage with, 85
  localization of, 7
  medulla oblongata, 109
  nontraumatic
    hypertension causing, 103
    images showing, 105-109
    vascular malformations and, 103-114

Hemorrhage(s), *cont'd*
  petechial, causing CT "fogging," 64
  posterior fossa, 107, 108
  punctate
    contrecoup, occipital fracture and, and diffuse axonal injury, 52-53
    trauma causing, 52-56
  subarachnoid; *see* Subarachnoid hemorrhage
  subdural
    hyperdensity with, 7
    subarachnoid hemorrhage with, 85
Hemorrhagic contusions, focal, 57
Hemorrhagic infarct, 64
Hemorrhagic metastases, 145, 146
Hemorrhagic tumor, subarachnoid hemorrhage caused by, 86
Herniation
  of anterior cerebral artery, 49
  rostrocaudal, 32
  subfalcial, chronic subdural hematoma with, 49
  tentorial, inability to identify basal cisterns and, 5
Herpes simplex encephalitis, 151, 154
Hounsfield, Sir Jeffrey, 1
Hydrocephalus, 5-6
  active, 6
  arrested, 6
  atrophy and, images showing, 157-164
  bacterial infections with, 150
  balanced, 6
  causes of, 5-6
  communicating, 5
  with intracerebral hemorrhage, 105
  noncommunicating, 5, 157-159
  nonobstructive, 5
  obstructive, 5, 32, 157-159
  shunt dysfunction with, 161, 162
  subarachnoid hemorrhage with, 85-86, 92, 93
  with third ventricle tumors, 118
  transependymal CSF flow in, 158
Hyperdense cerebral artery from infarction, 63
Hyperdense middle cerebral artery sign, 66-69
Hyperdense vessel sign with infarction in ACA and MCA territories, 74
Hyperdensities, abnormal, 7
Hyperperfusion after ischemic stroke, 64
Hypertension, nontraumatic hemorrhage caused by, 103
Hypodensity(ies)
  abnormal, 7-9
  fat droplets causing, 166
  from infarction, 63-64
    in ACA and MCA territories, 75
  radiation causing, 167
Hypoplasia
  frontal, 172
  temporal lobe, 172
Hypotension, systemic, watershed infarctions with, 65
Hypothalamus
  gliomas of, 117-118
  in middle-aged adult, 23
Hypoxemia, watershed infarctions with, 65

I

Infarct(infarction)(s)
    anterior cerebral artery territory, 73, 74-75
    basilar artery territory, 78-79
    brainstem, 80-81
    cerebellar hemisphere, 80
    cerebral, 6-7, 63-84
        gray matter hypodensities caused by, 8
    hemorrhagic, 64
    lacunar, 84, 166
    middle cerebral artery, 7
    middle cerebral artery territory, 66, 69, 70, 71, 74-75
        luxury perfusion with, 72
        subtle, 69, 70
    occipital lobe, 77, 78
        differentiating superior cerebellar cistern from, 190
    posterior cerebral artery territory, 78
    subacute, contrast obscuring, 4
    watershed, 65, 76
Infection(s)
    bacterial, 149-150
    chronic, 149
    intracranial, 149-156
        images showing, 151-156
    parasitic, 149
    TORCH, 149
    tuberculous, 150
    viral, 151
Inferior recess in middle-aged adult, 23
Injury, axonal, diffuse, occipital fracture and contrecoup punctate hemorrhage and, 52-53
Insula in normal young adult, 19
"Insular stripe, loss of," 7
    in ischemic stroke, 66, 67, 71
Interhemispheric fissure
    acute subdural hematoma in, 43
    in middle-aged adult, 24
    subarachnoid hemorrhage of, 89, 90
Internal auditory canal in normal young adult, 22
Internal capsule in normal young adult, 19
Internal carotid artery, 15
    in middle-aged adult, 23
Internal cerebral veins in normal young adult, 27, 28
Internal jugular vein, 13, 14
Internal occipital protuberance
    in normal young adult, 16, 19, 22
    streak artifact from, 41
Intra-axial metastases, 142-148
Intra-axial tumors, 116-117, 133-148
    CT characteristics of, 120
Intracerebral clot, frontal, acute, 93
Intracerebral hemorrhage, 105
    acute, 106
    contrast obscuring, 4
Intracranial air, occipital acute subdural hematoma with, 42
Intracranial hemorrhage, 94

Intracranial infections, 149-156
    images showing, 151-156
Intracranial neoplasms, 115-148
Intrahemispheric fissure, bifrontal contusions and acute hemorrhage in, 54
Intraparenchymal calcification, 169
Intraparenchymal hemorrhage
    intraventricular hemorrhage and, 107
    subarachnoid hemorrhage with, 85
Intraventricular hemorrhage
    intraparenchymal hemorrhage and, 107
    subarachnoid hemorrhage with, 85
Intraventricular pressure, raised, 5
Intraventricular tumors, 116
    CT characteristics of, 120
    differential diagnosis of, 116
    images showing, 128-132
Ischemia, 63
    white matter, white matter hypodensities caused by, 8
Ischemic stroke, 63-84
    images showing, 66-84

J

Jugular fossa in normal young adult, 22
Jugular vein, internal, 13, 14

L

Lacunar infarction, 84, 166
Large epidural hematoma, 32
Lateral ventricle
    in middle-aged adult, 23, 24, 25
    in normal young adult, 19, 20
Lentiform nucleus in normal young adult, 19
Leptomeningeal metastases, 127
Lesion(s)
    contrast enhancing, 4
    ring enhancing, 56
    space occupying, mass effect with, 5
Leukoencephalopathy
    atrophy and, 171
    from Binswanger's disease, 170
    multifocal, progressive, 155
Leukomalacia
    atrophy and, 171
    from Binswanger's disease, 170
    postradiation, 167
    white matter hypodensities caused by, 8
Level settings, 3
Line, orbitomeatal, 2
Lipomas, fat hypodensities caused by, 8
Lobe(s)
    frontal
        in normal young adult, 17, 21
        subarachnoid hemorrhage of, 91
    occipital, infarct of, 77, 78
        differentiating superior cerebellar cistern from, 190
    parietal, in normal young adult, 21

Lobe(s), *cont'd*
  temporal
    hypoplasia of, 172
    in normal young adult, 17
Loss
  of differentiation of gray-white interface, 8
    in diffuse cerebral anoxia postcardiac arrest, 165
    from infarction, 63, 71
  of "insular stripe," 7
    in ischemic stroke, 66, 67, 71
Lung, metastatic small cell carcinoma of, 142, 146
  with obstruction of aqueduct of Sylvius, 147-148
Luxury perfusion, 64
  of MCA infarct, 72
Lymphoma(s), 117, 138-139
  CT characteristics of, 120
  differentiation of, from glioblastoma multiforme, 137
  high grade glioma versus, 138

M

Macroadenoma, pituitary, 117
Macrophage activity causing CT "fogging," 64
Magnetic resonance imaging, CT versus, 1-2
Malformation(s)
  arteriovenous, 110-111, 112
    nontraumatic hemorrhage caused by, 104
    subarachnoid hemorrhage caused by, 86
  congenital, 178-180
  Dandy-Walker, 179
  dural, subarachnoid hemorrhage caused by, 86
  vascular
    images showing, 110-114
    nontraumatic hemorrhage and, 103-114
Mass effect
  with arachnoid cyst, 172
  diagnosis of, 5
  in herpes simplex encephalitis, 154
  from infarction, 63-64
  with posterior cerebral artery territory infarct, 78
  with tension pneumocephalus, 175
Mastoid air cells
  basal skull fracture through, 60-61
  in normal young adult, 16, 21
Mastoid sinuses, bacterial infections in, 150
Maxillary sinus in normal young adult, 16
Medium, contrast; *see* Contrast medium
Medulla oblongata
  hemorrhage in, 109
  in normal young adult, 16, 17
Medulloblastoma
  CT characteristics of, 120
  differentiation of
    from cerebellar astrocytoma, 132
    from intraventricular tumors, 116
"Medusa head" appearance with venous angiomas, 105
Melanoma, metastases from, 145
Meningeal carcinomatosis, 116

Meningeal deposits, nodular, 116
Meninges, metastases to, 125-126
Meningioma(s), 116, 121-122
  cerebellopontine angle, 118
  CT characteristics of, 120
  differentiation of, from supratentorial intraventricular tumors, 116
  suprasellar, 117
Meningitis
  bacterial, 150
  chemical, 8
  viral, 151
Metastases, 119
  extra-axial, 125-126
    CT characteristics of, 120
  hemorrhagic, 145, 146
  intra-axial, 142-148
    CT characteristics of, 120
  intraventricular, CT characteristics of, 120
  leptomeningeal, 127
  to skull or subjacent meninges, 125-126
  suprasellar, 117
Metastatic bronchoalveolar carcinoma, 143-144
Metastatic small cell carcinoma of lung, 142, 146
  with obstruction of aqueduct of Sylvius, 147-148
Middle-aged adult, normal brain anatomy of, noncontrast, 23-26
Middle cerebellar peduncle in normal young adult, 18
Middle cerebral artery, 15
  aneurysm of, 94, 95, 98, 101
    nontraumatic hemorrhage caused by, 104
    subarachnoid hemorrhage caused by, 94
  changes in, from ischemia, 63
  infarction of, 7
  in normal young adult, 26
Middle cerebral artery sign, hyperdense, 66-69
Middle cerebral artery territory infarct, 66, 69, 70, 71, 74-75
  luxury perfusion with, 72
  subtle, 69, 70
Middle cranial fossa
  acute epidural hematoma in, 36
  arachnoid cyst in, 172
  in normal young adult, 21, 22
Middle ear in normal young adult, 22
Midline abnormalities, 7
Mild atrophy, 164
  plagiocephaly and, with prominent subarachnoid space, 195
Mixed subdural hematomas, trauma causing, 57-62
Motion artifact, 177
MRI, CT versus, 1-2
Multifocal leukoencephalopathy, progressive, 155
Multiple sclerosis, advanced, 174
Mycotic aneurysm, 150
Myelinolysis, pontine, central, 168

N

Neoplasms
  contrast enhancing, 4
  intracranial, 115-148

Nerve, optic, in normal young adult, 16
Neurinoma, acoustic, 118, 124
    CT characteristics of, 120
Neuroanatomy, normal, 9-29
Neurocysticercosis, 149, 156
Nodular meningeal deposits, 116
Nodules of vermis in normal young adult, 18
Noncommunicating hydrocephalus, 5, 157-159
    subarachnoid hemorrhage with, 85-86
Noncontrast versus contrast cranial CT scans, 4
Nonobstructive hydrocephalus, 5
    subarachnoid hemorrhage with, 85-86
Nontraumatic hemorrhage
    hypertension causing, 103
    images showing, 105-109
    and vascular malformations, 103-114
Nontraumatic subarachnoid hemorrhage, 93
Normal structures, variations of, 177
    artifacts and congenital abnormalities and, 177-195
Nucleus
    caudate, in normal young adult, 19
    lentiform, in normal young adult, 19

O

Obstruction of aqueduct of Sylvius, metastatic small cell carcinoma of
    lung with, 147-148
Obstructive hydrocephalus, 5, 32, 157-159
    subarachnoid hemorrhage with, 85-86
Occipital acute subdural hematoma with intracranial air, 42
Occipital epidural hematoma, 35
Occipital fracture and contrecoup punctate hemorrhage and diffuse axonal
    injury, 52-53
Occipital horn in normal young adult, 20
Occipital lobe infarct, 77, 78
    differentiating superior cerebellar cistern from, 190
Occipital protuberance, internal
    in normal young adult, 16, 19, 22
    streak artifact from, 41
Oligodendrogliomas, 117, 134
Open lip schizencephaly, 179
Optic chiasm
    gliomas of, 117
    in normal young adult, 18
Optic nerve in normal young adult, 16
Orbit in normal young adult, 21, 22
Orbital roof in normal young adult, 22
Orbitomeatal line, 2
Ossification, 7
    of falx, 185

P

Paget's disease, 168
Papillomas, choroid plexus, differentiation of, from supratentorial intra-
    ventricular tumors, 116
Paranasal sinuses, bacterial infections in, 150

Parasitic infections, 149
Parietal contusion, 60-61
Parietal lobe in normal young adult, 21
Partial volume averaging effect, 177
Patient positioning for CT, 2
Peduncle, cerebellar, middle, in normal young adult, 18
Penumbra, 63
Perfusion, luxury, 64
    of MCA infarct, 72
Pericallosal artery in normal young adult, 27
Petechial hemorrhages causing CT "fogging," 64
Petrous apex in normal young adult, 22
Petrous bone beam hardening artifact, 194
Physics, CT, 2-3
Pineal gland in normal young adult, 19
Pineal tumors, 118
Pinna of ear in normal young adult, 16
Pituitary adenoma, 125
    CT characteristics of, 120
Pituitary fossa in normal young adult, 16
Pituitary macroadenoma, 117
Plagiocephaly and cortical atrophy with prominent subarachnoid
    space, 195
Plexus, choroid
    calcification of, 186-187, 193
    in middle-aged adult, 24
    in normal young adult, 19
Pneumocephalus, tension, 175
Pons in normal young adult, 17, 18
Pontine myelinolysis, central, 168
Porencephalic cysts, 179
Positioning, patient, for CT, 2
Postcentral sulcus in normal young adult, 21
Posterior cerebral artery, 15
    in normal young adult, 26
Posterior cerebral artery territory infarct, 78
Posterior communicating artery, 15
Posterior falx, chronic and acute subdural hematoma and, 46-47
Posterior fossa
    acute subdural hematoma in, 39
    hemorrhage in, 107, 108
Precentral gyrus in normal young adult, 21
Prepontine cistern, 10
    in normal young adult, 18
Pressure, intraventricular, raised, 5
Progressive multifocal leukoencephalopathy, 155
Prominence, sulcal, variation in, 191
Protuberance, occipital, internal
    in normal young adult, 16, 19, 22
    streak artifact from, 41
Pseudoporencephalic cysts, 179
Pseudotumor cerebri, 173
Punctate hemorrhage
    contrecoup, occipital fracture and, and diffuse axonal injury, 52-53
    and contusions, trauma causing, 52-56

Q

Quadrigeminal plate cistern, 10
  in normal young adult, 19
  subarachnoid hemorrhage of, 88

R

Radiation induced leukomalacia, 167
Recess, inferior, in middle-aged adult, 23
Reperfusion causing CT "fogging," 64
Ring enhancing lesion, 56
Rostrocaudal herniation, 32
Ruptured dermoid cyst, 166

S

Sac, aneurysmal, contrast enhancing, 4
Sagittal sinus, 13, 14
  in middle-aged adult, 24
  in normal young adult, 20, 28
  superior, venous thrombosis of, 81
  thrombosis of, 82
  variations of, 184
Scalp hematoma, air in, 60-61
Scanner, CT, 1
Scans, CT; *see* CT scans
Schizencephaly, 179
Sclerosis, multiple, advanced, 174
Scout view, 2
  use of, 5
Sella turcica, enlarged, 117
Septum pellucidum
  in middle-aged adult, 24
  in normal young adult, 19
Shunt dysfunction, 161, 162
Sigmoid sinus, 13, 14
Sign
  delta, 82
  hyperdense middle cerebral artery, 66-69
  hyperdense vessel, with infarction in ACA and MCA territories, 74
  star, 87, 88, 90, 93
  swirl, 33
Sinus(es)
  cavernous, 13, 14
  confluence of, 13, 14
  dural, venous thrombosis of, 83
  frontal, in normal young adult, 16, 21, 22
  mastoid, bacterial infections in, 150
  maxillary, in normal young adult, 16
  paranasal, bacterial infections in, 150
  sagittal, 13, 14
    in middle-aged adult, 24
    in normal young adult, 20, 28
    superior, venous thrombosis of, 81
    thrombosis of, 82
    variations of, 184
  sigmoid, 13, 14
  sphenoid, in normal young adult, 16, 21

Sinus(es), *cont'd*
  sphenoparietal, in middle-aged adult, 24
  straight, 13
    in middle-aged adult, 24
    in normal young adult, 20, 28
    variations of, 183
  transverse, 13, 14
    variations of, 183
  venous, 14
Skull
  "brass/beaten," 157, 158
  crooked, and cortical atrophy with prominent subarachnoid space, 195
  metastases to, 125-126
Skull base, fracture of, air collection caused by, 8
Skull fracture(s)
  basal, through mastoid air cells, 60-61
  basilar, air collection caused by, 8
  depressed, 60-61
  epidural hematoma caused by, 33
  frontal, contusion and, 55
  trauma causing, 31
Skull vault, fracture of, air collection caused by, 8
Small cell carcinoma of lung, metastatic, 142, 146
  with obstruction of aqueduct of Sylvius, 147-148
Space(s)
  CSF-containing, normal anatomy of, 9-13
  subarachnoid
    prominent, plagiocephaly and cortical atrophy with, 195
    variations of, 188-191
Space occupying lesion, mass effect with, 5
Sphenoid sinus in normal young adult, 16, 21
Sphenoid wing in normal young adult, 22
Sphenoparietal sinus in middle-aged adult, 24
Squamous cell carcinoma, 119
Star sign, 87, 88, 90, 93
Stenosis, aqueductal, congenital, 118
Straight sinus, 13
  in middle-aged adult, 24
  in normal young adult, 20, 28
  variations of, 183
Streak artifact, 177
  from internal occipital protuberance, 41
  in normal young adult, 18
"Stripe, insular, loss of," 7
  in ischemic stroke, 66, 67, 71
Stroke, ischemic, 63-84
  images showing, 66-84
Subacute infarction, contrast obscuring, 4
Subacute subarachnoid hemorrhage in basal cisterns, 5
Subacute subdural hematoma, 44
  density changes with, 44
  trauma causing, 44-51
Subarachnoid hemorrhage, 57
  acute, 91, 92, 93
  aneurysm of right middle cerebral artery causing, 94
  aneurysms and, 85-101

Subarachnoid hemorrhage, *cont'd*
   in basal cisterns, 5
   causes of, 86
   classic, 88-89
   contrast obscuring, 4
   CT interpretation in, 86
   images showing, 87-96
   noncontrast CT of, 11
   nontraumatic, 93
   normal CT scan differentiated from, 95
   subtle, 95, 96-97
   traumatic, 62
      trauma causing, 31
Subarachnoid space(s)
   effacement of, mass effect with, 5
   prominent, plagiocephaly and cortical atrophy with, 195
   variations of, 188-191
Subcortical arteriosclerotic encephalopathy, 170
Subcortical atrophy, 6
Subdural empyema, 150, 153
Subdural hematoma
   acute, 37-40, 57
      above tentorium, 40
      at tentorium, 62
      below tentorium, 39
      diffuse cerebral edema and, 58-59
      with evolution of contusion, 62
      from frontal to temporal parietal region, 37
      in interhemispheric fissure, 43
      occipital, with intracranial air, 42
      posterior falx and, 46-47
      in posterior fossa, 39
      subtle, 38
      trauma causing, 37-43
   acute on chronic, 45
      with fluid/fluid level, 50
   chronic, 47, 50-51
      posterior falx and, 46-47
      with subfalcial herniation, 49
      trauma causing, 44-51
   midline and, 33
   mixed, trauma causing, 57-62
   subacute, 44
      density changes with, 44
      trauma causing, 44-51
   suture lines and, 33, 37
   trauma causing, 31
Subdural hemorrhage
   hyperdensity with, 7
   subarachnoid hemorrhage with, 85
Subfalcial herniation, chronic subdural hematoma with, 49
Subtle acute subdural hematoma, 38
Subtle epidural hematoma, 34
Subtle middle cerebral artery territory infarct, 69, 70
Subtle subarachnoid hemorrhage, 95, 96-97
Sulcal prominence, variation in, 191

Sulcus(sulci)
   central, in normal young adult, 21
   effacement of, 6-7
      in MCA territory infarct, 71
   enlargement of, atrophy with, 163
   postcentral, in normal young adult, 21
Superior cerebellar artery, 15
Superior cerebellar cistern
   differentiating, from occipital lobe infarction, 190
   prominent, 189
Superior sagittal sinus
   in middle-aged adult, 24
   in normal young adult, 28
   venous thrombosis of, 81
Superior vermis
   in middle-aged adult, 23
   in normal young adult, 19
Suprasellar aneurysms, 118
Suprasellar cistern, 10
   in normal young adult, 18
Suprasellar meningiomas, 117
Suprasellar metastasis, 117
Suprasellar tumors, 117-118
Swirl sign, 33
Sylvian cistern in middle-aged adult, 23
Sylvian fissure
   in middle-aged adult, 23
   in normal young adult, 18
   subarachnoid hemorrhage of, 87, 88, 89, 90, 91, 93, 94
Sylvius, aqueduct of, metastatic small cell carcinoma of lung with obstruction of, 147-148
Systemic hypotension, watershed infarctions with, 65

T

Tectal gliomas, 118
Tectum in middle-aged adult, 23
Telangiectasias, capillary, nontraumatic hemorrhage caused by, 105
Temporal horn(s)
   dilated, 97
      subarachnoid hemorrhage and hydrocephalus with, 85-86
   in middle-aged adult, 23
   in normal young adult, 18, 27
Temporal lobe
   hypoplasia of, 172
   in normal young adult, 17
Temporoparietal region, acute subdural hematoma near, 37
Tension pneumocephalus, 175
Tentorial herniation, inability to identify basal cisterns and, 5
Tentorial vein in normal young adult, 27
Tentorium
   acute subdural hematoma above, 37, 40
   acute subdural hematoma at, 62
   acute subdural hematoma below, 39
   normal, 41
   variations of, 184

Third ventricle
    in middle-aged adult, 23
    in normal young adult, 18, 19
    subarachnoid hemorrhage of, 88, 89, 92
    tumors of, 118
Thrombosis
    dural sinus, 83
    sagittal sinus, 82
    venous, 81
Tissue densities, changing, 3
Tissues, appearance of, on CT, 3
Tonsil, cerebellar, in normal young adult, 17
TORCH infections, 149
Torcula, 13, 14
    in normal young adult, 27
    prominent, 188-189
    variations of, 183, 184
Toxoplasmosis, 149, 155
Transependymal flow of cerebrospinal fluid, 6
    in hydrocephalus, 158
Transverse sinus, 13, 14
    variations of, 183
Trauma, 31-62
    subarachnoid hemorrhage caused by, 86
Traumatic subarachnoid hemorrhage, 62
    trauma causing, 31
Tuberculomas, 150
Tuberculous infections, 150
Tumor(s)
    cerebellopontine angle, 118, 123
    contrast enhancing, 4
    CT characteristics of, 119, 120
    extra-axial, 116
        CT characteristics of, 120
        images showing, 121-132
    fourth ventricle, 116
        differential diagnosis of, 116
    hemorrhagic, subarachnoid hemorrhage caused by, 86
    hypodensities caused by, 9
    intra-axial, 116-117
        CT characteristics of, 120
        images showing, 133-148
    intraventricular, 116
        CT characteristics of, 120
        differential diagnosis of, 116
        images showing, 128-132
    pineal, 118
    suprasellar, 117-118
    of ventricles, 116

U

Unilateral watershed infarctions, 65

V

Variant, Dandy-Walker, 179
Variations
    of normal structures, 177
        artifacts, and congenital abnormalities, 177-195
    ventricular, images of, 192-193
Vascular malformations
    images showing, 110-114
    nontraumatic hemorrhage and, 103-114
Vascular structures, variations of, 181-184
Vascular territories, normal anatomy of, 15
Vein(s)
    cerebral
        internal, in normal young adult, 27, 28
        major, 14
    of Galen, 13
        in middle-aged adult, 24
        in normal young adult, 20
        prominent, 181, 182
        venous thrombosis of, 81
    jugular, internal, 13, 14
    tentorial, in normal young adult, 27
Venous angioma(s), 114
    nontraumatic hemorrhage caused by, 105
Venous confluence
    in normal young adult, 27
    prominent, 188-189
    variations of, 183, 184
Venous dural sinus thrombosis, 83
Venous sinuses, 14
Venous structures, normal anatomy of, 9, 14
Venous thrombosis, 81
Ventricle(s)
    asymmetry of horns of, 179
    congenital malformations of, 179
    effacement of, mass effect with, 5
    enlargement of
        atrophy with, 160, 163
            hydrocephalus causing, 6
    fourth; see Fourth ventricle
    lateral
        in middle-aged adult, 23, 24, 25
        in normal young adult, 19, 20
    normal anatomy of, 9-13
    third; see Third ventricle
    tumors of, 116
    variations of, images of, 192-193
Vermis
    nodules of, in normal young adult, 18
    superior
        in middle-aged adult, 23
        in normal young adult, 19

Vertebral artery, 15
    atheroma of, 186-187
    in normal young adult, 26
Viral infections, 151
Viral meningitis, 151
Volume averaging, 177

W

Watershed infarctions, 65, 76
White matter edema, white matter hypodensities caused by, 8
White matter hypodensities, 8

White matter ischemia, white matter hypodensities caused by, 8
Willis, circle of, 15
Window settings, 3

Y

Young adult, normal brain anatomy of
    contrast-enhanced, 26-28
    noncontrast, 16-22

Z

Zygomatic arch in normal young adult, 21